Concise
Oral Radiology

Second Edition

to

---

my wife, Vasu,
and
daughters, Medha and Anagha

Concise
Oral Radiology

Second Edition

HR Umarji

MDS (Oral Medicine and Radiology)

Professor and Head
Department of Oral Medicine and Radiology
Government Dental College and Hospital
Mumbai

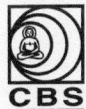

CBS

CBS Publishers & Distributors Pvt Ltd

New Delhi • Bengaluru • Chennai • Kochi • Kolkata • Mumbai
Hyderabad • Nagpur • Patna • Pune • Vijayawada

Concise **Oral Radiology**

Second Edition: 2011
Reprint: 2015, 2017

First Edition: 2008

Copyright © Author & Publisher

ISBN: 978-81-239-2008-5

Published by Satish Kumar Jain and produced by Varun Jain for

CBS Publishers & Distributors Pvt Ltd

4819/XI Prahlad Street, 24 Ansari Road, Daryaganj, New Delhi 110 002, India.
Ph: 23289259, 23266861, 23266867 Website: www.cbspd.com
Fax: 011-23243014   e-mail: delhi@cbspd.com; cbspubs@airtelmail.in.
Corporate Office: 204 FIE, Industrial Area, Patparganj, Delhi 110 092
Ph: 4934 4934   Fax: 4934 4935   e-mail: publishing@cbspd.com; publicity@cbspd.com

Branches

- **Bengaluru:** Seema House 2975, 17th Cross, KR Road,
  Banasankari 2nd Stage, Bengaluru 560 070, Karnataka, India
  Ph: +91-80-26771678/79   Fax: +91-80-26771680   e-mail: bangalore@cbspd.com
- **Chennai:** 7, Subbaraya Street, Shenoy Nagar, Chennai 600 030, Tamil Nadu
  Ph: +91-44-26680620, 26681266   Fax: +91-44-42032115   e-mail: chennai@cbspd.com
- **Kochi:** Ashana House, No. 39/1904, AM Thomas Road, Valanjambalam,
  Ernakulam 682 016, Kochi, Kerala, India
  Ph: +91-484-4059061-65   Fax: +91-484-4059065   e-mail: kochi@cbspd.com
- **Kolkata:** 6/B, Ground Floor, Rameswar Shaw Road, Kolkata-700 014, West Bengal, India
  Ph: +91-33-22891126, 22891127, 22891128   e-mail: kolkata@cbspd.com
- **Mumbai:** 83-C, Dr E Moses Road, Worli, Mumbai-400018, Maharashtra, India
  Ph: +91-22-24902340/41   Fax: +91-22-24902342   e-mail: mumbai@cbspd.com

Representatives

- **Hyderabad** 0-9885175004 **Nagpur**   0-9021734563   **Patna** 0-9334159340
- **Pune**   0-9623451994 **Vijayawada** 0-9000660880

Printed at Thomson Press India Ltd., Faridabad, Haryana, India

It is indeed a great pleasure in presenting this second edition of Concise Oral Radiology. It was gratifying to note that the first edition of this book was of much use for the undergraduate students preparing to face the examination. At the outset, Mr. Y.N. Arjuna, the Senior Director of CBS Publishers, suggested that various grammatical errors in the first edition should be corrected and appropriate addition or deletion should be carried out to make this book error-free. With this in mind the entire book was scanned for errors and additions such as introduction to CBCT, an appendix or differential diagnosis of radiographic appearances, etc. were made. The presentation of the book has also been improved upon to make it student-friendly.

I must thank Dr. Easwaran Ramaswamy, Dr. Amruta Bandal and Dr. Suvarna Sawant for their tireless efforts in improving upon the material of the first edition and I express deep appreciation to Mr. Y.N. Arjuna who inspired and guided us to do the best.

HR Umarji

Preface to the First Edition

Ideals are like little stars, We cannot reach them
But we benefit by their presence.

— *John Le Carre*

No claim is made regarding the originality of the text in **Concise Oral Radiology**. In fact the idea behind this publication was to present important aspects of oral radiology available in various standard textbooks in a nutshell so as to help the undergraduate students, too hard pressed for time, to refer to many textbooks.

I have drawn heavily on the knowledge, experience and teachings of great stalwarts in oral radiology in India, Dr GJ Merchant, Dr AB Surveyor, Dr Jakhi, D Ani John, Dr BK Parikh and Dr RN Mody. Under their guidance I have learnt this subject. These stalwarts permitted me to sit near their feet, but should not be blamed for my simplicity.

The efforts required to publish a book, however concise, was too cumbersome for a lazy man like me, too skeptical of his knowledge. Dr. Easwaran Ramaswami, however, did not have the shortcomings of his teacher and spared no efforts to accomplish the task. I shall be forever grateful to him for all his help and tireless efforts.

There is always a need for a detailed and in-depth study of any topic and for such reasons the reference books are mentioned at the end of the chapters. To maintain the text brief and succinct, I have been ruthless in slashing large portions of information and may also be accused of oversimplification. Despite these and several other shortcomings, I venture to hope that this text will not make an unwelcome or unworthy addition to an ever-increasing list of textbooks in the subject of oral radiology.

I am indeed fortunate to be associated with Government Dental College and Hospital (GDC & H), Mumbai, as a student and a teaching staff and my contributions in this text (radiographs, etc.) are only because I happened to work in this great institution and collected the material from the patients attending GDC & H OPD. I have always felt encouraged in this institute and feel proud to belong to it.

I have been constantly encouraged and inspired by the students of GDC & H (both undergraduate and postgraduate) and the staff members. I am indebted to them as I have learnt so much from interactions with them.

I am also grateful to Miss Jyoti Madaan for excellent art work and Mr. Balram Solanki and BR Sharma of CBS Publishers and Distributors for all their help.

HR Umarji

Contents

CHAPTER 1

Introduction and Basic Radiation Physics

Definitions

Radiology is defined as the study and use of radiant energy including Roentgen rays, radium and radioactive isotopes as applied to medicine and dentistry.

Roentgenology is the study and use of Roentgen rays as applied to medicine and dentistry.

Radiography is the production of a photographic image of an object through the use of X-rays.

Radiation is the process of transfer of energy from one point to another in the form of electromagnetic waves, e.g. light, radio waves, X-rays,.

Matter is the substance of which all physical things are composed, it is anything that occupies space and has inertia, it has mass and can exert force and can be acted upon by a force. Matter can exist in three states, viz. solid, liquid and gaseous.

Atom is the fundamental unit of any particular element. It has central nucleus of protons and neutrons and negatively charged electrons orbiting around it. (*A* means *cannot, tomi* means *to cut.*)

Atomic number is the distinguishing number of protons in the nucleus of an atom and is designated by the symbol Z.

At rest position, number of electrons is equal to the number of protons.

Atomic mass number denotes the total number of protons and neutrons, in the nucleus, and is designated by the symbol A.

Discovery of X-rays

On the night of 8th November 1895, Prof. Wilhelm Conrad Roentgen, who was a professor of Physics at the University of Wurtzberg, Germany, accidentally discovered X-rays. He was experimenting with Hittorf-Crookes tube for cathode rays, when he observed a greenish glow emanating from barium platinocyanide screen kept at a distance. When he interposed his hand, unintentionally, between the tube and the screen, he could detect the image of his bones in the shadow. He at once realized the significance of this finding and established the property of penetration. He then covered the tube with black paper and fluorescence persisted, which further confirmed the property of penetration. He also realized that this new kind of a ray must be responsible for fogging of photographic plates observed by him, and reported by others (photographic property).

Roentgen had discovered these new rays and as anything unknown in mathematics is designated by symbol 'x', he called them X-rays. His colleagues described this as an un-American modesty, and they later insisted on calling X-rays as Roentgen rays.

The first radiograph was made immediately afterwards and was of his wife Bertha's hand. The exposure time required was 15 minutes!

The first dental X-ray was made by **Otto Walkhoff.** The exposure time was 25 mins!

The first intraoral X-ray was made by **Dr. Edmund Kells** in 1896.

Unfortunately, early workers failed to realize the harmful effects of X-rays, who worked without protection and suffered from skin ulcerations, necrosis and even malignancies and underwent mutilating surgeries. Only **Sir Rollins** had realized the possibility of radiation hazards and had advised certain precautions to be taken to prevent them and hence he is known as the "Father of radiation protection".

Radiation is the transfer of energy from one point to another in the form of waves or movement of particles. Particulate radiation consists of alpha and beta rays. Alpha rays are positively charged and they are made up of 2 protons (He nuclei). Beta rays are nothing but a stream of electrons.

Electromagnetic radiation which includes the various rays mentioned in the Table 1.1 is explained on the basis of two theories:

1. Wave theory
2. Quantum theory

PROPERTIES OF ELECTROMAGNETIC (EM) RADIATION

1. It travels in a straight line by wave motion.
2. While passing through matter EM radiation gives rise to two fields: a magnetic field at right angles to pathway of propagation, and an electric field at right angles to magnetic field.
3. The basic difference between various electromagnetic radiations is in their wavelengths.

Table 1.1: Electromagnetic spectrum		
Type of rays	*Wavelength*	*Required potential difference in kVp*
Electric Waves	10^{18}Å (50000–100,000 kHz)	
Hertzian Waves	10^{13}–10^{18}Å (1000 kHz)	
Radio/Wireless/TV	10^{10}–10^{12}Å (1–100 kHz)	
Infrared	10^5 Å	
Visible Light Red	7700 Å	
Violet	4000 Å	
Ultraviolet	1000Å	
Grenz rays	1.2 Å	10–20 kV
Soft X-rays	0.5–1Å	20–50 kV
Diagnostic X-rays	0.1–0.5 Å	500–100 kV
Therapeutic X-rays	0.01A–0.05Å	200–500 kV
Supervoltage/Megavoltage	0.001Å	2–20 meV
Cosmic X-rays	0.0001Å	

Å = Angstrom unit

4. All EM radiations travel at the speed of 3×10^8 m/s or 1,86,000 miles per second (speed of light).
5. They can travel through vacuum.
6. Exhibit phenomena of diffraction and interference.
7. Follow the inverse square law;

$$\text{Intensity } \alpha \ \frac{1}{\text{Distance}^2}$$

Visible light has wavelength between 4000 and 7000 Å; violet has a shortest wavelength (4000Å) and red has the longest wavelength (7000 Å).

UV light has shorter wavelength than violet light. It produces following effects on skin:

1. Photoerythema (sunburn)
2. Photopigmentation (suntan)
3. Photochemical production of vitamin D

It can also be used for sterilization of eatables and other substances and treatment of skin lesions such as psoriasis and PUVA therapy for lichen planus.

Electromagnetic waves which have still shorter wavelength (0.1 to 0.5Å) make them more penetrating and these are the X-rays used for diagnostic purpose.

EM radiations used for radiotherapy should have still shorter wavelength (0.01–0.001Å) and greater penetration and capacity to kill malignant cells.

Electromagnetic radiations having longer wavelengths than red are called infrared rays and are the part of sunlight manifested as heat. They are also used to relieve painful muscle spasm.

Radio waves having wavelengths (10^{10}–10^{11} nm) are used in magnetic resonance imaging (MRI)

Uses of X-rays

1. Diagnostic
2. Therapeutic – X-rays have capacity to damage the living cells which are rapidly multiplying and therefore cancer cells are more prone to damage by X-rays.
3. In metallurgy – crystallography
4. Spectroscopy – identification of certain substances
5. Sterilization of tinned foods
6. Detection of casting defects in metallic objects.

CONSTRUCTION AND WORKING OF X-RAY MACHINE

Principle

Electric energy can be converted into kinetic energy (potential difference can be used to give speed to electrons). Kinetic energy of electrons can be converted into heat and X-rays.

The X-ray tube is a highly evacuated glass tube (lead beryllium glass) in which are mounted cathode and anode assembly (Fig. 1.1). The X-ray tube is evacuated because:

(i) Presence of air will obstruct flow of electrons and reduce their kinetic energy

(ii) Presence of oxygen will oxidize the tungsten filament.

The lead beryllium glass is surrounded by lead (Pb) shield except in the area of the port. Lead shield is used because:

(i) It absorbs all the radiations except the useful beam.

(ii) It provides earthing to the X-ray tube to prevent chances of electric shock

(iii) Prevents physical damage to the tube.

Cathode is made up of tungsten (symbol W) filament mounted in the concavity of molybdenum focusing cup.

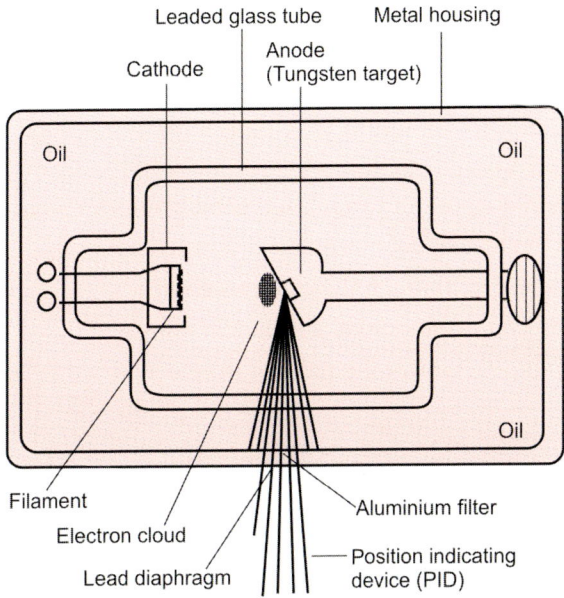

Fig. 1.1: Construction of X-ray tube.

Tungsten is preferred as a filament material because it has:

1. High atomic number (z = 74) therefore more number of electrons are given out, i.e. high thermionic emission.
2. High melting point (3380°C) so that filament should not melt.
3. Low vapour pressure at high temperature so that it will not vaporize.

Tungsten filament is in the form of a coil 1 cm in length and 0.2 cm in width, mounted on 2 stiff wires.

The function of molybdenum focusing cup is to restrict the size of electron cloud and also serve as a cathode and help in repelling electrons (because of negative charge).

The anode is made up of tungsten button (focal spot or target) mounted in a copper stem. Tungsten is preferred as a target material because it satisfies the requirements of ideal target material, i.e.

1. High atomic number (Z =74); which gives rise to increased interactions between incoming electrons and tungsten atoms thereby generating more number of X-ray photons.
2. High melting point (3380°C) so that anode does not melt, despite the heat produced there.

3. Low vapour pressure at high temperature, so that tungsten does not evaporate. Such vapours if present are likely to line the tube and give rise to excessive filtration and also act as a source of radiation giving rise to stray radiations.

However tungsten does not have good thermal conductivity and hence it is mounted in copper stem which is a good conductor of heat.

The heat generated at the anode is dissipated by:

1. *Conduction:* through the copper stem.
2. *Convection:* through oil surrounding the tube.
3. *Radiation:* through the radiator device attached to copper stem.

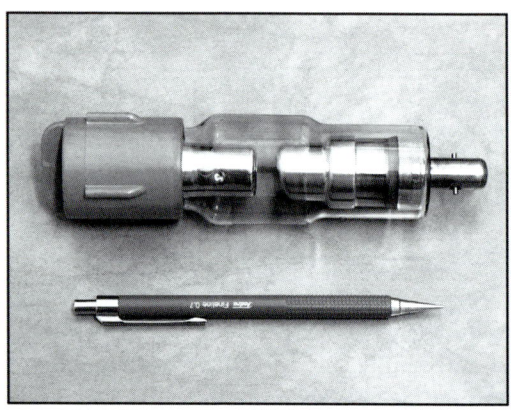

Fig. 1.2: X-ray tube.

THE WORKING OF X-RAY MACHINE

When electrons traveling at a high speed are suddenly stopped by an impact against a solid object, X-rays are produced. In an X-ray machine, electrons are produced, by heating the filament electrically. An electron cloud is produced at the cathode by thermionic emission. Size of the electron cloud is restricted by molybdenum focusing cup. These electrons will travel at high speed only when anode is made positive. This is done by applying a potential difference of 65,000 volts between anode and cathode. As the anode is made positive with respect to the cathode the electrons present around the filament are strongly repelled from cathode and they are bombarded against the focal spot where X-rays are produced along with heat. 99.8% of the kinetic energy (KE) is converted into heat which is dissipated as stated above and only 0.2% is converted into X-rays. X-rays so produced are allowed to come out through the port of the X-ray tube.

Interaction between Incident Electrons and Atoms of the Focal Spot

Characteristic Radiation

When electrons approach the tungsten anode, if kVp is more than 70 then K-shell electron is knocked off and L-shell electron falls in its place. In doing so, L-shell electron gives out energy which is equivalent to difference of energy level between K and L shells. This energy is in the form of X-radiation and since energy level of a particular element at each shell is characteristic, the radiation given out is called as ***characteristic radiation*** (Fig. 1.3).

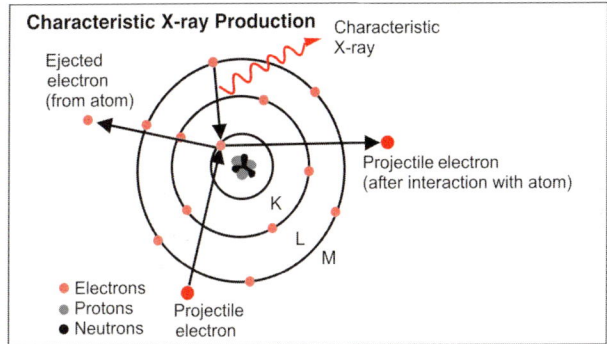

Fig. 1.3: Production of characteristic radiation.

Braking Radiation or Bremsstrahlung

When kVp is less than 70, incoming electrons undergo a sudden change in direction and sudden reduction of speed, i.e. they decelerate (because they are repelled by electrons of tungsten atom). Due to this change in speed of the electrons, the radiation which is given out is known as braking radiation and also called as white radiation. Mostly the radiations generated in a dental X-ray machine are of this type (Fig. 1.4).

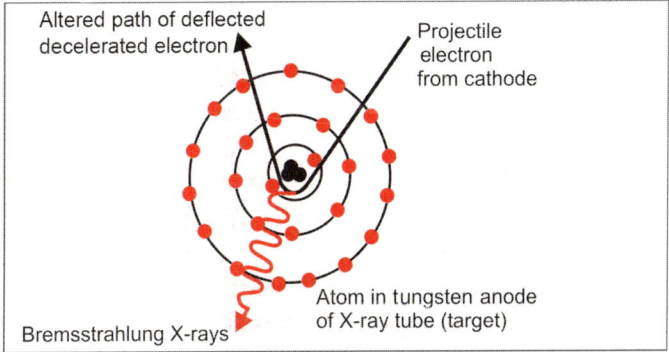

Fig. 1.4: Production of braking radiation.

Circuit of X-ray Tube (Fig. 1.5)

It is divided into two parts:

1. Filament circuit (to produce electrons by heating filament).
2. Cathode-Anode circuit (to provide the potential difference of 65,000 volts).

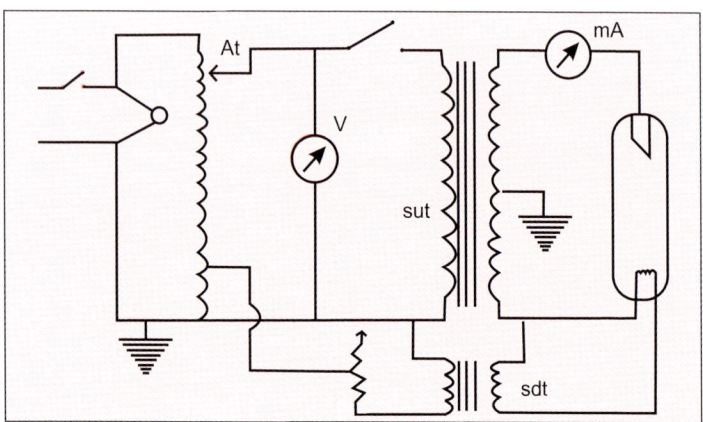

Fig. 1.5: Circuit diagram of X-ray tube mA : Milliammeter, V : Voltmeter, At : Auto transformer, sut : Step up transformer, sdt : Step down transformer.

Filament circuit uses a step down transformer (sdt), because, only 10 V is required to heat the filament, whereas supply is 220 V.

Cathode-anode circuit has a step-up transformer (sut) because the voltage has to be stepped up from 220V to 65,000V.

Auto-transformer which has a kVp selector is used to regulate kVp to a certain degree and it has a single coil which is divided by means of a pointer.

A *step-down transformer* has less turns of coil in the secondary as compared to the primary.

In the *step up transformer* the number of turns of coil in the secondary are more compared to primary.

Line Focus Principle: Angle of Truncation

The actual size of focal spot is 1 mm × 3 mm. However, the anode is angled at 20 degrees to central ray, as a result of which the rectangular focal spot appears as a square (Fig. 1.6). This is done to facilitate the following:

(i) Heat distribution across larger surface (less heat per unit area) at the anode and at the same time.

(ii) Sharp image because rectangular focal spot appears as a square when viewed in the direction of the central ray (smaller the focal spot sharper the image).

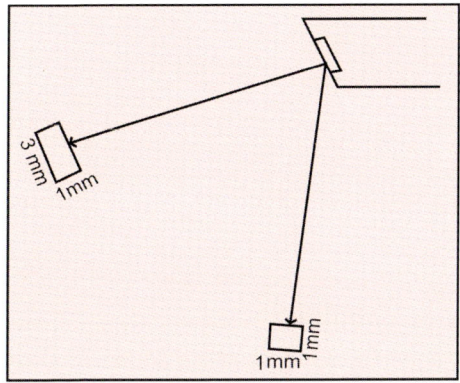

Fig. 1.6: Diagram explaining the line focus principle.

Heel Effect

The intensity of the emergent beam is not uniform because a part of the X-ray beam is absorbed by the focal spot itself. If the anode was not angulated and was flat, the 'Heel' of the target would have absorbed most of the X-ray photons. The cathode side of the beam is more intense as it does not have to travel through the target as much as the anode side of the beam which gets absorbed in the target itself and this contributes to 'heel effect'.

Rotating Anode

In certain machines, anode is in the form of a copper disc 7.5–10 cm in diameter. Focal spot is in the form of 0.6 mm ring incorporated in copper disc. During exposure, the copper disc is rotated so that at each moment a different part of focal spot gets bombarded by electrons (Fig. 1.7). This gives rise to less heat per unit area.

Milliamperage

Milliamperage (mA) denotes the current which is supplied to the filament. If mA is increased, the temperature of the filament also increases, thereby increasing thermionic emission. This gives rise to greater number of electrons striking against anode and as a result more number of X-ray photons. Thus mA controls the quantity of X-rays. The number of X-ray photons will also increase if the exposure time is increased.

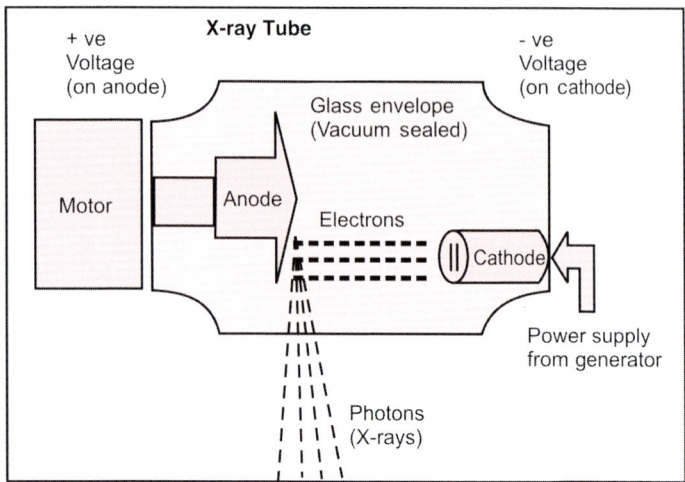

Fig. 1.7: Diagram showing a rotating anode. (Source : Internet)

mAS factor (milliamperes × seconds): denotes product of mA and exposure time in seconds. If mAS is increased more number of X-ray photons are produced. In other words, mAS factor, denotes total photon production and mAS controls quantity of X-rays.

kVp (kilovoltage peak) denotes potential difference between cathode and anode. If kVp is increased, the electrons travel at a greater speed and have a greater KE. As a result more interactions take place within the focal spot hence more X-ray photons of short wavelength are given out. The energy of the X-ray photons is related to the kinetic energy of incoming electrons and therefore if kVp is increased the penetration power of X-rays increases.

Rectification is the conversion of alternating current (AC) to direct current (DC). During the first phase of the AC cycle, the cathode is negatively charged and anode is positively charged. The electrons hit against the anode and X-rays are produced. But when current changes its direction during the second phase, cathode becomes positively charged. Therefore electrons present at anode (because of the thermionic emission secondary to the heat produced), travel backwards and hit against the filament, thereby causing burnout of the filament. Such a phenomenon takes place in a general X-ray machine where high kVp is used. Hence, a rectifying device such as a diode or a triode valve is used to rectify the direction of the current.

In a dental X-ray machine, however, the amount of heat produced at the anode does not give rise to excess electrons. As a result, when current changes its direction, there are no electrons at the anode to travel back to the cathode and hence dental X-ray tube is called as *self rectified*.

Primary radiation is the radiation emitted by the focal spot of the target.

Stray radiation is the radiation emitted by any part of the X-ray tube other than the focal spot.

Useful beam is that part of primary radiation which is allowed to emerge out through the collimating device.

Scattered radiation is the radiation which has undergone a change in direction during passage through a substance.

Secondary radiation is the radiation emitted by a substance through which X-rays are passing.

PROPERTIES OF X-RAYS

1. Diagnostic Properties

A. Penetration

(a) X-rays can penetrate through matter in a differential manner. Degree of penetration of X-rays depends on the kVp of the X-ray machine. It varies inversely as wavelength and directly as kVp. For diagnostic radiography wavelength used is 0.1 to 0.3 Å.

(b) Penetration of X-rays also varies according to density of material through which they are passing, e.g. penetration is more through pulp, less through dentin and lesser through enamel because the density of enamel is more (Inorganic content, i.e. Ca–96%).

(c) Penetration also depends on the thickness of material through which they are passing.

B. Photographic Properties

X-rays can produce photochemical reaction of sensitized surface of the film. When X-rays pass through a film at a particular point, certain changes occur in Ag-Br crystals at that point which when developed appear as dark shadows known as a radiolucent shadow, e.g. pulp, whereas enamel does not permit more X-rays to pass through and hence appears as white this is called radiopaque.

C. Fluorescence

When X- rays fall on certain crystalline substances they emit visible light, e.g. barium platinocyanide gives rise to green light. Calcium tungstate gives blue light and the recently used (rare earth materials) gadolinium and lanthanum give rise to greenish fluorescence.

2. Biological Properties

X-rays can have harmful effect on living cells, as X-rays can directly damage the DNA, chromosomes and also other cellular components. Such genetic changes can have a cytocidal effect on the cells and this is termed as the **direct effect** of radiation. Sometimes repeated exposure to X-rays may cause formation of a "mutant gene" which may lead to carcinogenesis.

Indirect effect of radiation is associated with formation of unstable compounds, alteration of the cellular enzymes, etc. with which the body cells are incompatible.

3. Thermal Properties

When X- rays pass through matter they give rise to heat, however, it is very negligible.

4. Chemical Properties

Since X- rays are ionizing radiations, they can cause alteration in the chemicals through which they pass, e.g. $FeCl_2$ to $FeCl_3$, H_2O to H^+ and OH^-.

5. Properties of Physics

1. X-rays are invisible electromagnetic radiations.
2. They travel at the speed of light, i.e. 1, 86,000 miles/sec or 3×10^8 meters/sec.
3. They cannot be focused.
4. They obey the laws of polarization and interference.
5. They satisfy the *"inverse square law"*, i.e. intensity of X-ray beam at a given point varies inversely as square of the distance of that point from the source of radiation (focal spot).

FACTORS AFFECTING THE RADIOGRAPHS

There are three basic points common to all the radiographic procedures and these are the X-ray source, the patient and the film or other image receptors. Any variation in these can alter the radiograph and hence the factors are divided as follows,

    I. Radiation beam factors (X-ray source)
   II. Object factors (Patient/Object)
  III. Image recording factors (Film)

I. Radiation Beam Factors

1. *Focal Spot Size*

If the size of the focal spot is large each point on the focal spot acts as source of X-rays and the rays incident on the object cast the shadow at different spots giving rise to unsharpness or penumbra formation (e.g. your shadow under a tube light appears to be unsharp). If the source is small, the shadow becomes sharper (e.g. your shadow under a light bulb appears to be sharp). Therefore, it is said that the focal spot should be as small as possible to obtain a very sharp image (Fig. 1.8). Ideally, a point source should be used but it is not practically possible and hence we use a focal spot which is 1 mm × 3 mm rectangular which is projected as a square (line focus principle).

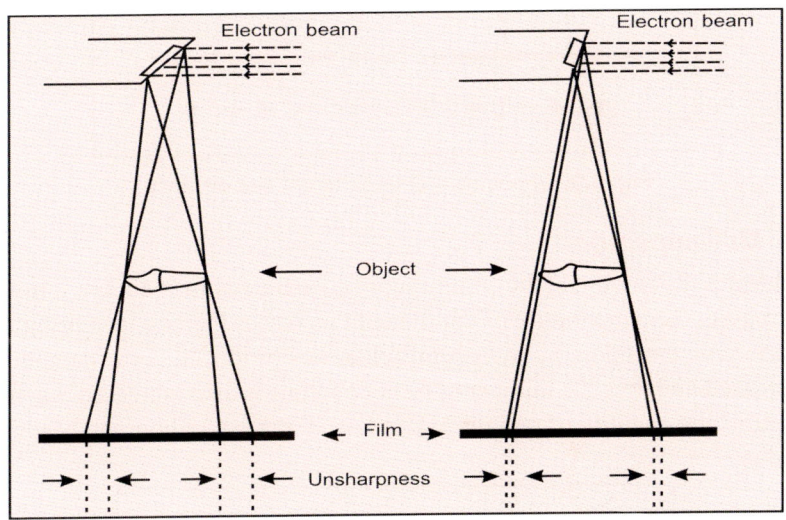

Fig. 1.8: Diagram showing the importance of a point source.

2. *Target Film Distance (TFD)*

TFD should be as long as possible. As X-rays coming from a distance are more parallel and less divergent, there is less magnification and penumbra formation (Fig. 1.9). However, TFD cannot be increased indefinitely because of the inverse square law. Thus each technique has its own ideal TFD, e.g.

1. Periapical radiographs
   – Bisecting angle technique – 6 to 8"
   – Paralleling technique   – 16 to 18"
2. Cephalometric projection – 5 feet
3. Other extraoral views   – 3 feet

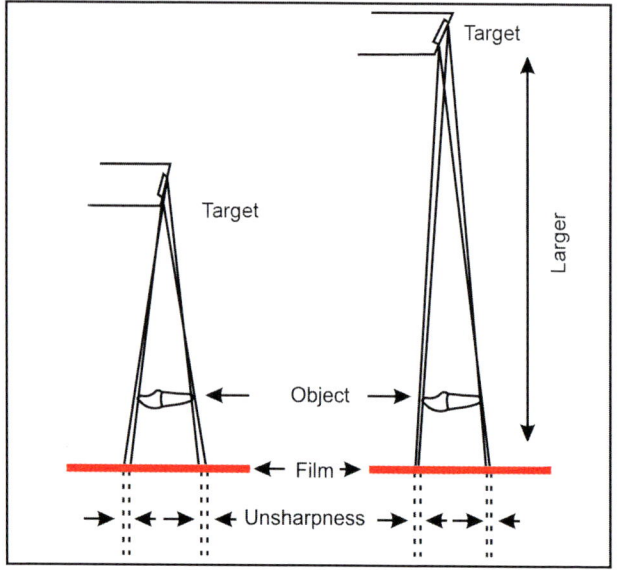

Fig. 1.9: Importance of large target film distance.

3. *Milliamperage*

It denotes the amount of the current supplied to the filament circuit. If mA is increased, the temperature of the filament increases thereby increasing the thermionic emission, i.e. number of electrons produced at the cathode is increased and thus the number of X-ray photons is also increased, i.e. mA controls the quantity of radiation. If mA is increased, radiograph becomes darker.

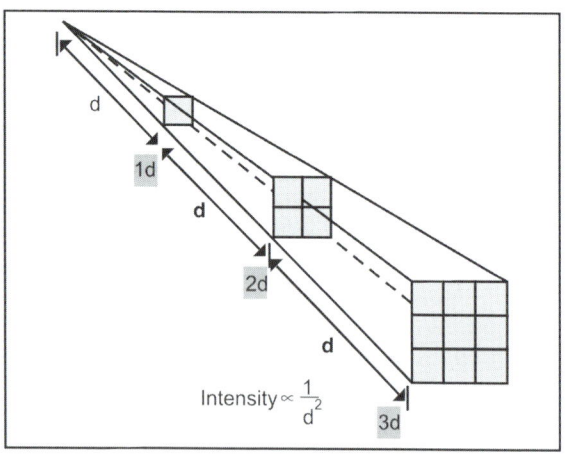

Fig. 1.10: Inverse square law.

4. *Kilovoltage Peak (kVp)*

It denotes the potential difference between the anode and the cathode. If kVp is increased the K.E. of the electrons increases and this gives rise to more penetrating X-ray photons, i.e. kVp controls the quality of radiation. Increased kVp also increases the mean energy of the photons, maximum energy of the photons and also increases the number of photons as a result of increased number of interactions between incident electrons and target atoms. However, kVp cannot be increased indefinitely because all X- rays might pass through the object without being absorbed, giving rise to a very poor contrast. On the other hand, if kVp is too less the resultant beam of X-rays will have a very less penetrating power and will be entirely absorbed by the object. Each technique requires an optimum kVp, e.g.

1. Periapical radiographs – 65 kVp,

2. PA Waters, Paranasal view –70 kVp.

5. *Filtration*

Since the kVp across the tube varies from 0–65,000 V the X- ray photons which come out are not of uniform wavelength. Therefore the X-ray beam is made up of long wavelength photons or soft X-rays and short wavelength photons or hard X-rays. The soft X-rays do not penetrate the hard tissue structures and they are fully absorbed in the tissues, causing harm. Short wavelength photons, i.e. hard X-rays on the other hand have the capacity to penetrate the tissues and cast a shadow and hence are of use in diagnostic radiography. The purpose of filtration is to eliminate or to cut off long wave photons and this is achieved by the following means:

    (a) Inherent filtration   – Glass wall of X-rays tube.

                                        – Oil surrounding the X-ray tube.

                                        – Cone of the tube.

    (b) Added filtration: 1.5 to 2.5 mm thickness. Aluminium disc is an added filter.

    (c) Total filtration: Sum total of inherent and added filtration is known as total filtration.

6. *Collimation*

Is the restriction or controlling the size and shape of the X-ray beam so as to avoid damage caused by radiation. The collimating device helps us to expose only the area to be imaged as it restricts the size and shape of the

X-ray beam and protects the adjacent structures against radiation exposure and damage.

Collimation can be achieved by:

(i) *Lead (Pb) diaphragm*, which is 2 mm thick, in which there are number of apertures. The Pb diaphragm is adjusted for obtaining a suitable beam size. If the aperture is round, the resultant beam is cone-shaped. If the aperture is rectangular, the resultant beam is pyramidal. The diameter of the circular beam at the skin level should be 2¾th of an inch.

(ii) *Pb lined cylinders:* Nowadays open ended Lead lined cylinders are preferred. Such cylinders further restrict the X-ray beam size from the open end.

(iii) *Slit beam collimators* of dimension 2 mm × 30 mm are used in OPG machines to produce a slit beam which substantially reduces the radiation exposure to the patient. The OPG machine also utilizes *post-patient collimation* in the form of metallic sheet in front of the cassette which has a slit permitting the X-rays to pass through to reach the cassette.

7. Tube Rating

These are specifications that show the operating limits of the X-ray tube, i.e. maximum exposure time for which the tube may be energized without damage to the target from overheating at a particular kVp and mA.

8. Duty Cycle

It relates to how frequently successive exposures can be made without damage to the tube, and depends on the heat build up, i.e. kVp × mA × sec.

II. Object Factors

1. Object Density

A dense structure has the capacity to absorb more number of X-ray photons than a relatively less dense structure. As a result of this, dense structures appear radiopaque or white (enamel or silver filling, etc.) whereas, less dense structures (dentine, cementum, etc.) appear comparatively less radiopaque, while the pulp or periodontal ligament space allows maximum number of X-ray photons to pass through and hence will appear darkest (radiolucent). Thus, the density of an object plays an important role in diagnostic radiography and at times exposure factors have to be modified to obtain a good X-ray picture.

2. *Object Thickness*

If the object to be radiographed is thicker then kVp or penetration power of the X-ray is to be increased along with exposure time to obtain a good radiograph. Thicker objects also have a greater disadvantage because they may generate more scattered radiation which in turn gets absorbed by the object thereby increasing radiation damage.

III. Image Recording Factors

1. *Reduction of Secondary and Scattered Radiation*

(a) *Pb foil* is used in intraoral film packet for the following reasons:

X-rays which have passed through the film are of no further use in diagnostic radiography. On the contrary, they can irradiate the tissues behind the film and this can also result in scattered or secondary radiation capable of travelling backwards (back scatter) thus leading to fogging of the film.

The lead foil used in the X-ray film packet.

   (i) Absorbs the X-rays which have passed through the film and reduces the patient exposure.

  (ii) Absorbs the back scatter and prevents fogging of the film.

 (iii) Gives stiffness to the film packet.

The lead foil has a typical pattern to it, e.g. tyre track, herring bone, etc. Whenever the film is placed wrongly this pattern appears on the film and this reverses the side identification as the embossed dot does not face the tube.

(b) *Pb backing* of the cassette: Similar functions are served by it because it absorbs the back scattered X-rays as well as those that have passed through the film.

2. *Grids*

When a beam of X- rays passes through an object it gets split into 2 types of photons:

   – Forward moving primary photons, which are carrying the message to the film.

   – Obliquely moving scattered photons, which are likely to cause fogging of the film as they have changed their direction.

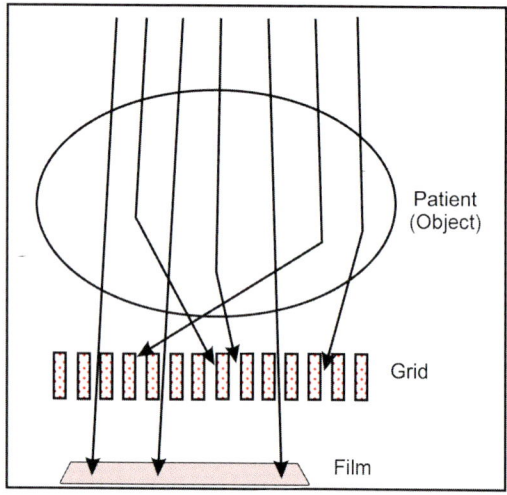

Fig. 1.11: Diagram explaining the principle of a grid.

The purpose of the grid is to cut off the obliquely moving scattered photons (Fig. 1.11). Grid is a sheet of radiolucent material in which are incorporated strips of lead (Pb). As the Pb strips are parallel the scattered photons moving obliquely strike the lead strips at an angle and are absorbed by them and only the forward moving primary photons which are relatively straight are allowed to pass. The grid is used in extraoral radiography and is placed between the object and the film.

Types of grids:

(a) *Stationary Grids*

    (i) **Linear/Parallel grid:** Pb strips are placed parallel to each other. In this type at the periphery the divergent primary photons may get cut off and therefore the grid has to be modified.

   (ii) **Focused grid:** In this type, to eliminate primary photons being cut off at the periphery, Pb strips are focused towards the X- ray source (Fig. 1.12).

  (iii) **Pseudo-focused grid:** In this type, there is a progressive diminution in the height of the Pb strips from the centre to the periphery. As the strips are shorter at the periphery the primary photons are allowed to pass (Fig. 1.13).

  (iv) **Crossed grid:** To eliminate the X-ray photons which are scattered in the plane of Pb strips, 2 grids are placed at right angles to each other, known as crossed grid.

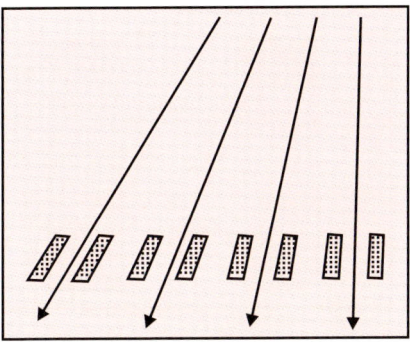

Fig. 1.12: Arrangement of lead strips in a focused grid.

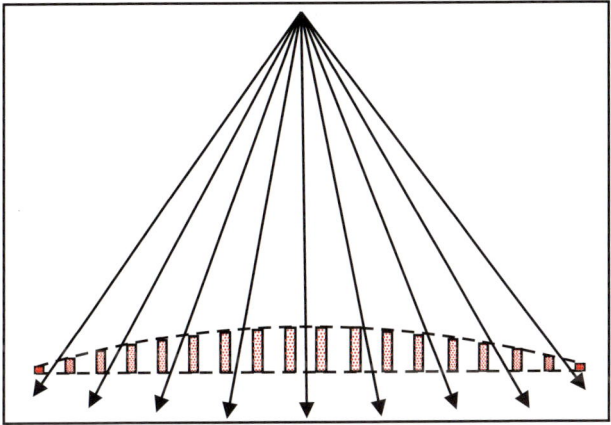

Fig. 1.13: Arrangement of lead strips in a pseudo-focused grid.

(b) *Movable Grid/Potter-Bucky diaphragm:* If a stationary grid is used the rays are absorbed by the Pb strips and white lines appear on the film. This can be eliminated if the grid is moved at a regular speed during the exposure. Such movable grids are called Potter-Bucky diaphragm.

GRID RATIO is given by the formula

$$r = h/D,$$

Where   r   =   grid ratio

        h   =   height of lead strips

       D   =   distance between two adjacent lead strips

            (Fig 1.14).

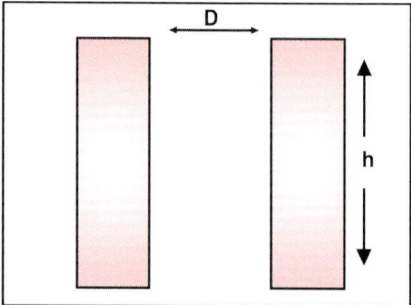

Fig. 1.14: Measurements for the calculation of grid ratio.

It indicates the efficiency with which the scattered photons are absorbed. The disadvantage of using a grid or Potter-Bucky diaphragm is that the exposure time has to be increased as the Pb strips absorb the X-ray photons and reduce the number of incident photons.

3. *Films and Film Storage*

In olden days the films were made of glass plates wrapped in black paper and rubber dam material to prevent leakage of saliva. After that cellulose nitrate base was used, but this has two main disadvantages:
  – Cellulose nitrate base is highly inflammable and
  – Films used to curl.

This was overcome by the use of cellulose triacetate. Recently, polyester base and polyethylene terephthalate is used.

Construction

Film is made up of two components (Fig. 1.15):

(a) A *Base* which is 0.2 mm thick and is made up of polyethylene terephthalate or cellulose triacetate.
   – It has transparent bluish tint.
   – Its function is to provide uniform support to the emulsion.

(b) *Emulsion*: It consists of silver halide (bromide and iodide) crystals suspended in a gelatinous/ non-gelatinous matrix which acts as a vehicle. This vehicle keeps the silver halide crystals evenly or uniformly dispersed. During film processing the vehicle absorbs the processing solutions thereby allowing the chemicals to react with the silver halide crystals. The silver iodide crystal has a larger diameter and disrupts the regularity of the Ag-Br crystal and increases the sensitivity of the Ag-Br.

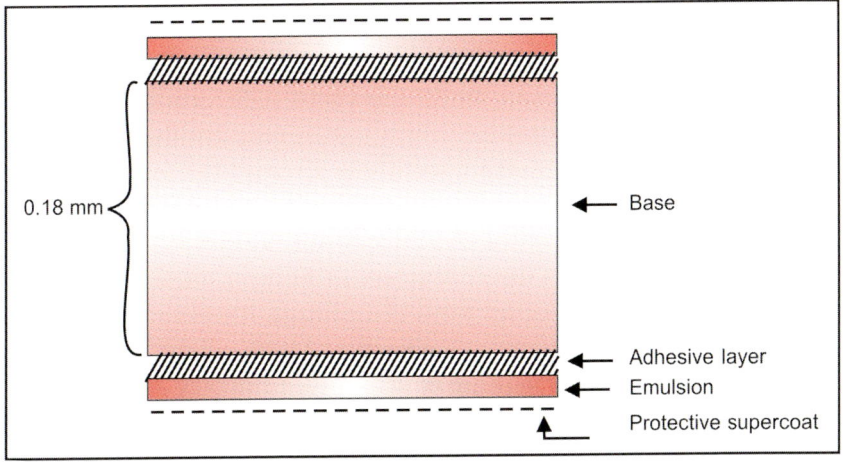

Fig. 1.15: Composition of a film.

- Thickness of the emulsion is 0.01 mm and it is present on both the sides of the transparent base thereby increasing the radiosensitive material and reducing the exposure time.
- It is sensitive to light and X-rays.
- It is the active component of the film.

In between the emulsion and the base there is an adhesive layer. The emulsion is covered with protective super coat (a dense layer of gelatin).

This coat protects the film during handling and from the rollers during automatic processing.

The film packet contains

1. An outer packet made up of a sealed *plastic cover* to prevent ingress of light and saliva. The side of the film packet which is to touch the teeth and face the X-ray tube is usually white and has a pebbled (older films) or smooth surface. The reverse side of the film has usually two colors, e.g. blue and white or black and white to help prevent wrong placement of the film and has a triangular flap to help strip the film packet

2. Inside the film packet there is a *black envelope* covering the film which protects the film from light and damage during removal from the packet.

3. *Lead foil*

4. *Film*

I. *Films are Classified As*

1. *Screen and* 2. *Non-screen*

    1. Screen films are more sensitive to visible light because colour dyes are added to the emulsion, which make it more sensitive to particular light given out by the intensifying screens. The green sensitive dyes added to the surface of tabular grains increase their light gathering capacity. The absorbing dye in the emulsion also prevents crossover of light from one screen to the other side emulsion. This helps to prevent unsharpness of the image. It is essential to use the proper film and screen combination. Mostly all the films used in extraoral radiography are of screen type and they are used along with intensifying screens provided in specialized containers called *Cassettes*.

    2. Non-screen films do not have special dyes added to their emulsion and they are sensitive to X-rays. Mostly all the intraoral films are of non-screen type. (Exception: Upper true occlusal wherein intraoral cassette with correct screen film combination is used.) Non-screen films are of the following types:

    (a) Periapical film

    (b) Occlusal film

    (c) Bite wing film

II. *According to Speed*

If exposure time required to produce a radiograph of useful density is less then it is called as a fast speed film. The speed of film depends on:

    (a) Grain size: The size of Ag halide grains. The larger the size of the crystal the faster is the speed.

    (b) Thickness of emulsion: Thicker the emulsion more is the radiosensitive material available and faster is the speed.

But larger the grain size lesser is the sharpness of the film, which affects the details of the film. To overcome this T-mat G films were introduced wherein the grain is flat or broad at the film surface and narrow towards base (like letter T) so that film speed can be increased without compromising the sharpness of the image.

Insight film utilizes tabular grains of mean diameter 1.8 mm and ultra speed film -1 mm. The tabular grains are oriented parallel with film surface and offer large cross-sectional area to the X-ray beam hence 'Insight film' requires half as much exposure as an ultra-speed film. According to speed the films are of the following types:

1. Speed A
2. Speed B
3. Speed C
4. Speed D
5. Speed E/ Ekta speed.

III. *According to their size*

1. Periapical size O = 22 × 35 mm, size 1 = 24 × 40 mm, size 2 = 31 × 41 mm
2. Bitewing : 31 × 41 mm
3. Occlusal: 57 × 76 mm
4. Orthopantomograph: 6 × 12" (15 cm × 30 cm)
5. Lateral oblique: 5 × 7"
6. PA Waters/mandible; lateral cephalogram, etc. : 8 × 10"

PROPERTIES OF FILMS

1. **Density** is defined as the degree of blackness present on the film measured in terms of light transmission on a logarithmic scale, e.g. if a beam of light is filtered to its 1/10th by a film then density is 1 and if a beam of light is filtered to its 1/100th then its density is 2. The density of an ideal diagnostic film should be 0.1 to 0.2. Density of the film depends upon the exposure time and mA and it is directly proportional to these factors. The relation of density to the log of exposure is given by the characteristic curve (H-D curve)

2. **Contrast** is the difference in the various gradations of density in the different areas of a radiograph. If between total white and total black there are very few areas of varying densities then it is called a *high contrast* or *short scale* contrast gradation. If between the total white and total black there are more number of areas of varying densities it is called as *low contrast* or *long scale contrast* gradation.

   Contrast is related to kVp of the beam. If kVp is increased the contrast decreases and vice versa. However, for each radiographic technique one must employ adequate kVp and obtain optimum contrast to make the relevant details fully apparent.

   Factors influencing the contrast:

(a) Milliamperage and exposure time (mAS)

(b) Kilovoltage peak (kVp)

(c) Filtration

(d) Object thickness and density

3. **Detail** is the ability of the radiograph to reproduce the sharp outlines. It depends on:

   – Size of Ag-Br crystals, smaller the size of the crystal, better and sharper are the details.
   – Focal spot size.
   – Movement of the patient.

4. **Latitude** is a measure of range of exposures that can be recorded as series of distinguishable densities on the film. Wide latitude means long scale contrast gradation. By increasing the kVp, the latitude increases.

5. **Mottle** appears as areas of uneven density on exposed radiograph visualized as darker and lighter areas on the film.

   The factors influencing mottle are:

   (a) Film graininess, becomes obvious with magnification.

   (b) Use of intensifying screens increases the mottle.

6. **Resolution**: It is the ability of the radiograph to record separate structures that are close to each other. It is measured by calculating the Line Pairs per mm. For OPG it is 5 line pairs per mm and for IOPA it is 10 line pairs per mm. Factors such as focal spot size, film grain size, patient movement which affect 'detail' also affect the resolution.

   Parallax error: As the films used routinely are double emulsion films and the X-ray beam is divergent, there is a certain degree of unsharpness. This happens because the shadow of the point on the object is recorded at different spots by the 2 sides of the emulsions. This is normally not discernible. But if the film is wet and hence the emulsion swollen, the image may appear unsharp.

Storage of X-Ray Films

While storing films one must avoid light, heat, electricity, moisture and sources of radiation. In other words, X-ray films are to be stored in a cool, dry place away from sources of radiation in lightproof containers.

Intensifying Screens

These are used in extraoral radiography to reduce exposure time. Intensifying screens intensify the action of X-rays (on the film) by converting the X-ray photons into visible light by the property of fluorescence. It is made up of 4 layers:

- Plastic base or polyester base.
- Reflecting layer (Titanium dioxide).
- Active phosphor layer, which contains fluorescent material.
- Protective super coat.

Active phosphor layer is made up of calcium tungstate which emits blue light, or rare earth materials such as terbium activated gadolinium oxysulphide ($Gd_2O_2S : Tb$) and thulium activated lanthanum oxybromide ($LaOBr : Tm$) which emits green light. The construction of a cassette having intensifying screens is shown in Figure 1.16.

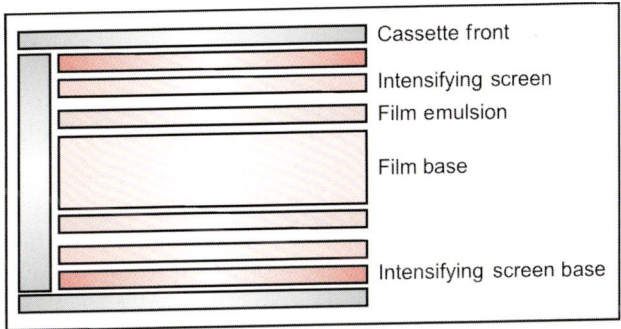

Fig. 1.16: Cross-section of a cassette with intensifying screens.

Functions

By utilizing the property of fluorescence the intensifying screen converts X-rays into visible light. As a result of this the X-ray film placed between the 2 intensifying screens in the cassette gets exposed not only to X-rays but also to visible light produced by both the screens. Intensifying screens thus intensify the action of X-rays and reduce the exposure time. The front screen in thin to provide adequate penetration to X-ray photons. The back screen is thick to capture majority of the X-ray photons.

Speed of the intensifying screens: If exposure time required to produce a radiograph of useful density with a particular screen is less, then the speed is said to be fast. The speed of the intensifying screen depends upon:

- The size of the fluorescent crystals, i.e. larger the size, faster the speed.

– Thickness of the phosphor layer, i.e. thicker the layer, faster the speed.

However, if the speed of the intensifying screen is more, then the sharpness decreases, because of larger crystal size. For example, OPG film appears unsharp compared to IOPA because hi-speed film and screen is used in OPG.

Sharpness is defined as the ability of the film to define an edge precisely, e.g. DE junction, trabecular pattern.

Radiographic Blur or Unsharpness is because of:

(a) Image receptor blurring

(b) Motion blurring

(c) Geometric blurring

Image receptor blurring can be because of:

(i) Double emulsion film causing parallax error, more apparent when film is wet.

(ii) Large grain size of fast speed film.

(iii) Large grain size of the intensifying screen: Visible light and ultraviolet radiation emitted by the screen spreads out beyond the point of origin and expose the film area larger than the phosphor crystal causing unsharpness. Thicker phosphor layer causes dispersion of light and hence blurring. It is important to maintain a very close contact between screen and film to minimize unsharpness caused by dispersion of light and to maximize image sharpness.

When intensifying screens are used, parallax distortion contributes to image unsharpness. This happens because light from one screen may cross the film base to reach the emulsion on the opposite side. This problem can be solved by incorporating dyes in the emulsion to absorb the emitted light.

PROPERTY OF IONIZATION

When X-ray photons pass through matter, one of the following four things can happen:

1. X-ray photons pass through matter without any change in the photon or in the matter.

2. X-ray photons may cause vibrations of the electrons in the atoms of matter, which return to their own shell. This phenomenon is called EXCITATION, coherent or elastic scattering.

3. Sometimes, photons may displace an electron. In doing so it may lose a little of its energy and will emerge out as a scattered photon (with change in its direction). This is called COMPTON EFFECT/SCATTER.

4. Sometimes, it may displace centrally located K or L shell electrons. The electron in the adjacent shell falls immediately in the vacant shell. In doing so, it liberates energy equivalent to the energy difference between the two orbits/shells. Since the energy level at each shell for a particular element is characteristic. The energy given out in the form of radiation is called as CHARACTERISTIC RADIATION. Because complete energy of the X-ray photon is utilized to displace the inner shell electron and because the photon displaces an electron, this is called as PHOTOELECTRIC EFFECT.

Thus Compton Effect is good for the patient as it is less hazardous but bad for the film production as it contributes to unwanted fogging. The vice versa is true for photoelectric effect, which is less hazardous for the image production, but bad to the patient as it results in greater exposure.

FILM PROCESSING

At the microscopic level the silver halide crystal shows distribution of the Ag^+, Br^-, I^- and relatively free interstitial Ag^+ ions. An unexposed film contains Ag, Br, I in ionic (charged) form. There is an important site present at the periphery termed as Latent Image Site containing sulphur impurity (Triallyl carbamide), which can capture the electrons and help in precipitation of Ag.

LATENT IMAGE PRODUCTION (Fig. 1.17)

When an X-ray photon passes through Ag halide crystal it knocks off an electron from the Br ion and liberates an electron. (Two such neutral Br atoms joint together to form Br gas which is liberated in the emulsion.)

$$Br^- + X\text{-ray} \longrightarrow Br + e^-$$
$$Br + Br \longrightarrow Br_2 \uparrow$$

Electrons liberated by Br ion are captured at the site known as LIS (latent image site) which is sulphur impurity within the crystal (Triallyl carbamide).

Interstitial Ag ions which are positively charged and relatively free traverse through the crystal and accumulate in these latent image sites to

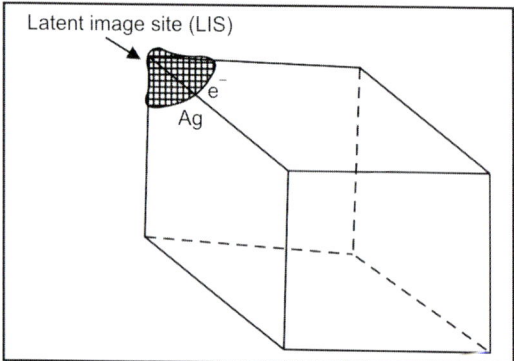

Fig. 1.17: Latent image site in the crystals.

form a neutral silver atom. Thus, millions of specks of silver are formed in an exposed X-ray film and are collectively called as latent image. The formation of latent image disturbs the ionic status of the crystal and makes it vulnerable to the electrons donated by the developer. When the film is immersed in the developer, metallic silver gets deposited in those crystals in which latent image is formed. During fixing, the unexposed Ag^+ and Br^- crystals are dissolved by the fixing agent.

DEVELOPER

The developer contains the following constituents:

1. Developing agent:
   (a) Elon/Metol or phenidone, which produces the details by donating electron to the silver ions and causing them to precipitate.
   (b) Hydroquinone, which provides the contrast.
      Phenidone donates electrons to the silver bromide in the emulsion and when exhausted hydroquinone supplies electrons to phenidone.

2. Restrainer: Potassium bromide (KBr) or benzotriazole. It acts as an anti-fog agent and prevents the developing of the unexposed crystals.

3. Activator: Sodium bicarbonate. It provides the alkaline medium (pH = 7+) which is required for the emulsion to swell up and open the pores so that the developing solutions can pass into the emulsion and can bring about the precipitation of silver.

4. Preservatives: Sodium sulphite. It prevents the oxidation of the developing agent because it has comparatively a greater affinity for oxygen. It forms a colorless soluble compound with the oxidized developer, thereby preventing yellowish brown stains on the film.

5. Vehicle: Water in which all the constituents are mixed.

FIXER

The fixer contains the following constituents:

1. **Clearing Agent:** The clearing agent used is ammonium thiosulphite. This removes the undeveloped silver halide crystals thereby clearing the film. Failure to remove these crystals makes the radiograph dark and non-diagnostic.

2. **Acetic Acid:** It acts as buffer to maintain the pH of about 4 to 4.5. This acidic environment is required to achieve good diffusion of the clearing agent into the emulsion. It also helps to stop the developing process thereby preventing continued development of unexposed crystals.

3. **Hardener:** The hardener used is potash alum. This helps to harden the gelatin which has been softened during developing.

4. **Preservative:** Preservative used is sodium sulphite ammonium sulfite. It forms a colorless soluble compound with the oxidized developer which is carried over to the fixer, thereby preventing yellowish brown stains on the film.

5. **Vehicle:** Water in which all the constituents are mixed.

PROCESSING

It is a collective title given to a series of procedures carried out in the dark room namely: Developing, Rinsing, Fixing, Washing, Drying

METHODS OF PROCESSING

1. **Time temperature method:** In this method, the temperature of the developer is controlled at 68°F and the films are developed for 5 minutes. A special timer is provided which will give out a signal at the end of 5 minutes.

Advantages

(i) If at 68°F, the films are dark, it implies that the films are overexposed. In other words, it means that this method maintains a direct check on the exposure time.

(ii) It is the most standardized procedure and does not require expertise as opposed to the visual method.

Disadvantage

Unlike the visual method, the films cannot be overdeveloped or underdeveloped to obtain the desirable contrast.

2. **Visual method:** In this method, the films are held against the safe light from time to time during development. The moment the pulp chamber becomes evident or the roots are seen separate from the bone, developing is said to have completed.

Advantages

(i) If the X-ray film is overexposed, it can be underdeveloped and vice versa to obtain the derived density.

(ii) X-ray film can be developed to obtain the desirable contrast, e.g. Films can be underdeveloped to see the hypocalcified salivary calculus and buccal/lingual expansion of cyst or tumors.

Disadvantages

(i) It is not a standardized procedure.

(ii) It requires expertise and experience.

3. **Modified time temperature method:** A special chart can be prepared mentioning the developing time at a particular temperature, taking into account the age of the developing solution in number of days.

4. **Daylight processing:** This is carried out in a special device having safe light filters and two gloves like compartments through which the operator can put his hands and develop the films. The process obviates the need for a dark room.

5. **Automatic processing:** A special roller system is provided into which the film is fed. Developing, fixing and drying takes place as the film passes through the roller system. A fully processed and dry film is made available within the shortest possible time. Such a unit is ideal for urgent radiographs. Certain automatic processors have a web system instead of a roller. The processing chemicals

of these systems are maintained at a suitable higher temperature to ensure rapid developing and effective hardening materials such as glutaraldehyde is added in the developer itself.

6. **Monobath:** The film packet is itself provided with a developer and fixer and the X-ray films can be developed on the spot. A dark room is not required. It is ideal for root canal treatment where urgent radiographs are required or in places where dark room facilities are not available.

IMPORTANCE OF RINSING

Blister formation/pitted radiograph:

1. If the film is not rinsed prior to fixing, the developer is carried on to the fixer and neutralization reaction takes place. Sodium bicarbonate reacts with the acetic acid in the fixer to liberate carbon dioxide gas which gives rise to blister formation in the emulsion. These blisters then rupture giving rise to a pitted radiograph.

2. **Dichroic fog:** If the developer is carried to the fixer, it reacts with the silver thiosulphate present in the fixer and causes precipitation of silver on the film. This results in fogging which appears as pink in transmitted light and green in reflected light. Hence this is called as dichroic fog.

IMPORTANCE OF FIXING

If the films are not fixed adequately, the unexposed AgBr crystals remain on the film which when exposed to light can turn brown/black thereby making the film useless. The ideal fixing time is 15–20 minutes. To confirm that the fixing is adequate, the film is viewed in bright light and it is ascertained whether the light transmission is complete in the most radiopaque region.

IMPORTANCE OF WASHING

During fixing, the AgBr crystals are dissolved in the fixer and two types of silver thiosulphates are formed: the soluble and insoluble form. The soluble form dissolves in the fixing tank. This insoluble form remains adherent to the film and if not washed out in running water, it gets exposed to light and atmosphere giving rise to yellowish brown stains on the film. The adherent silver thiosulphate can only be removed by washing the film under running water for at least 15 minutes.

THE DARK ROOM

The dark room for processing the films must have the following requirements.

1. Developing tanks for the developer, fixer and running water, an inlet and outlet for water.
2. A dry working table for handling the films prior to developing.
3. Cupboard for storage of the films.
4. The entrance to the dark room may be in the form of a maze or a labyrinth or must have a door which can be bolted from inside.
5. *Illumination:* The dark room must be fitted with a bright tube light for use during non working hours. Safe lights illumination must be provided for use during film developing. Red bulbs of 10–15 watt with ruby red filter can be used with one bulb fitted above the developing tanks, one above the working table and one on the ceiling. The minimum distance between the table and the red light must be 4 feet. The Kodak GBX2 filter bulbs can also be used safely in the dark room.
6. *Ventilation:* The room should be airconditioned and should have two fans: one for inlet for fresh air and one exhaust fan located at a higher level to drive out the foul air.
7. Cleanliness and tidiness are very important in the dark room and everything should be kept in its proper place.

SUGGESTED READING AND REFERENCES

1. Oral Radiology. Principles and Interpretation: White and Pharoah—5th edition.
2. Essentials of Dental Radiography and Radiology—Eric Whaites, 3rd edition.
3. Fundamental Physics of Radiology—Meredith, Massey.

CHAPTER 2

Radiobiology

Radiobiology is the study of the effects of ionizing radiation on biological tissues. Ionizing radiation can cause as well as can be used to diagnose and treat malignant neoplasms.

While using ionizing radiation for diagnostic radiography, we have a responsibility to ourselves, our progeny as well as patients and neighbours. People who operate X-ray machines are called as *occupationally exposed persons.*

When X-rays pass through matter, one of the following things can happen:

(a) Majority of the times no change takes place within the matter or the X-ray photon.

(b) The low energy photon may interact with the outer shell electron to vibrate momentarily. The incident photon ceases to exist and a scattered photon of the same energy and frequency is emitted at a different angle from the path of the incident photon (***elastic scatter***).

(c) Electrons are knocked off and the X-ray photons lose their energy to continue as a long wave scattered photon. This effect is called as ***Compton effect.***

(d) K-Shell electrons may be knocked off and the complete energy of the photon is absorbed by the matter. Since, in this effect, a high speed electron is given out by the photon, it is called as the ***photoelectric effect.***

(e) **Pair production:** If the kVp is more than 70, the photon splits into one positron and one electron (Pair production). The positron which is a highly reactive positive electron combines with an electron and produces two photons which travel in opposite direction (***Annihilation radiation***).

In short, passage of X-rays through matter gives rise to electrons which travel through the matter. These electrons keep on causing ionization and can give rise to damage to biological tissues. An electron can cause:

– ionization
– excitation
– breaking of chemical bonds

LINEAR ENERGY TRANSFER (LET)

It is the measure of energy released by the ionizing particle (such as a high speed electron). As LET increases, the biological effect of radiation increases. As the electron moves along its track, it decelerates till it comes to a stop. The LET increases with the decrease in the speed of the electrons. This relation between the speed of the electrons and the linear energy transfer is referred to as *Bragg effect*.

Radiation Effects can be Classified as

(A) 1. Direct
     2. Indirect

    1. ***Direct effect:*** The energy of the photon or secondary electron is directly transferred to the biological macromolecule causing damage.

    2. ***Indirect effect:*** The energy of the photon or secondary electron brings about the ionization of water and the formation of H^+ and OH^- ions (radiolysis of water) which are known as *free radicals*. These free radicals will combine with each other in an abnormal way, e.g. two molecules of water will split to give rise to a molecule of hydrogen and a molecule of hydrogen peroxide. This gives rise to molecules which are not compatible with the body cells because, 75% of the cells are made up of water. Thus more damage is caused by the indirect method.

Radiation effect can also be classified as Somatic and Genetic.

(B) 1. Somatic
     2. Genetic

    1. ***Somatic effect:*** It is the effect of ionizing radiation on the cells of the body, other than the gamete producing cells giving rise to biological harm evident in one's own lifetime.

2. *Genetic effect:* It is the effect of ionizing radiation on the reproductive cells which are damaged and hence the defect is manifested in the progeny, e.g. stillbirth, miscarriage, aneuploidy; missing, malformed or excessive limbs.

The cellular component most vulnerable to radiation damage is DNA and the damage is more evident during its replication. DNA is a double helix of sugar and phosphate compound with adenosine, guanine, cytosine and thiamine and this forms a unit of a gene.

The effects of radiation can be in the form of (Fig. 2.1):

(i) Base damage
(ii) Single chain break
(iii) Double chain break
(iv) Inactivation of repair enzymes.

Normally the changes in the DNA are cytocidal, but sometimes, the genetic damage persists and is transmitted in the next generation.

Irradiation of the cell after DNA formation results in damage to the single arm known as **chromatid aberration** while irradiation before DNA formation has taken place results in damage of both the arms known as **chromosome aberration**.

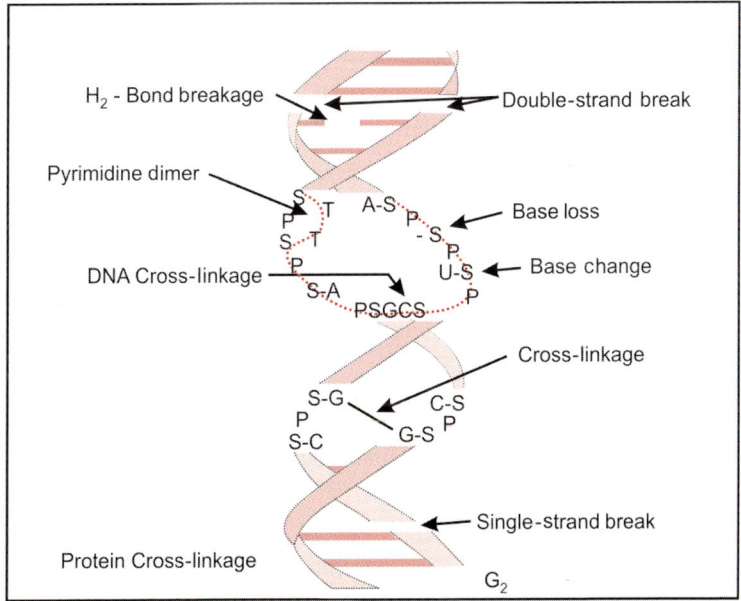

Fig. 2.1: Radiation damage to DNA.

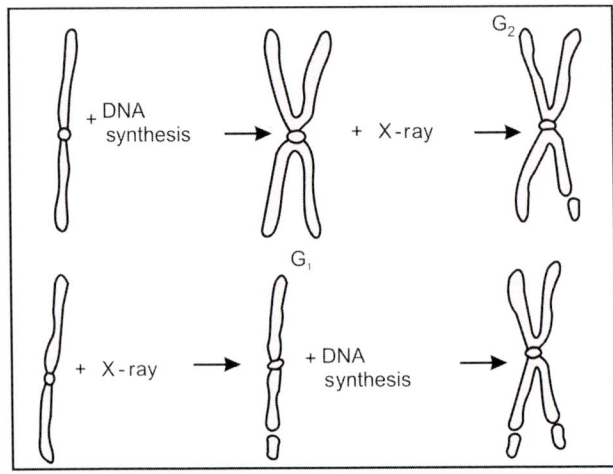

Fig. 2.2: Chromatid aberration (above) and chromosome aberration (below).

(C) *Biologic effects* of ionizing radiation may be divided into two broad categories:

    1. Stochastic effect

    2. Deterministic effect

    1. **Stochastic effects:** Stochastic effects are all or none effects for which the probability of occurrence rather than the severity depends on the radiation dose received, e.g. radiation induced cancer.

    2. **Deterministic effects:** Deterministic effects are those in which the severity of the radiation induced damage depends upon the dose of radiation received, e.g. radiation mucositis.

The effect of radiation depends upon:

    (a)   Dose response relationship

    (b) Tissue variability

    (c) Area of radiation

    (d) Latent period

    (e) Individual variation

Dose response relationship: This may be of the following types:

    1. Linear type or

    2. Non-linear type

    1. **Linear type:** Here in this type, if the dose is increased the response goes on increasing, e.g. cataract formation.

2. **Non-linear type:** Till a particular dose limit is reached, no response takes place, e.g. radiation induced erythema.

Tissue Variability

Certain tissues are more susceptible to ionizing radiation than other tissues, mainly the cells undergoing rapid division. Cells which are stable and which are highly differentiated undergo less radiation damage. The susceptibility in a decreasing order is as follows:

- Blood forming and reproductive cells.
- Young bone, glandular tissue and GIT epithelium.
- Skin and muscles.
- Nervous tissue (CNS) and adult bone.

Most radiosensitive cells are the ones which undergo many future mitosis, have a high mitotic rate and are in a primitive stage of differentiation. This is called the ***Bergonie and Tribondeau law.*** Figure 2.3 shows the stages of cell cycle.

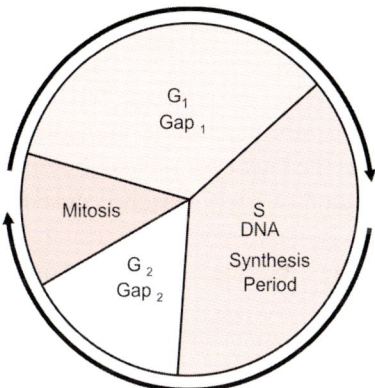

Fig. 2.3: Cell cycle.

Based upon the radiosensitivity, mammalian cells are classified in five types. They are:

1. Vegetative intermitotic cells
2. Differentiating intermitotic cells
3. Multipotential connective tissue cells
4. Reverting postmitotic cells
5. Fixed postmitotic cells.

Based upon the radiosensitivity, the body cells can be divided into three types (Table 2.1)

Table 2.1: Relative radiosensitivity of various organs

High sensitivity	Intermediate sensitivity	Low sensitivity
• **Lymphoid organs**	• **Fine vasculature**	• **Mature RBC**
• Bone marrow	• Growing cartilage	• Optic lens
• Intestinal lining cells	• Growing bone	• Muscle cells
• Basal cells of oral mucous membrane	• Salivary glands	• Neurons
• Germ cells of the testis		

Area of Radiation

Based upon the area of body which receives the radiation, two types of effects are noted, i.e. specific area radiation and whole body radiation.

Whole body radiation (WBR) is more harmful than specific area radiation. In diagnostic radiography WBR is relevant to the fetus, as even if the mother receives specific area radiation, for the fetus, it can be WBR more so if the fetus is small.

Latent Period

The effect of radiation is not manifested immediately, but after a certain period. This is called as the latent period and may vary from a few days to a few weeks. The duration of latent period is dose related. At supra lethal doses, i.e. more than 5 Gy, it extends from few hours to few days, but at sub lethal doses, i.e. less than 2 Gy, the latent period may last longer up to few weeks.

Individual Variation

Some individuals are more susceptible than others and so our responsibility is to protect the weakest and therefore the tolerance dosage and safety dosage should be determined with a view to protect even the weakest individual.

Radiation Hazards

These may be manifested during one's lifespan or in the future generation (shortening of lifespan, genetic harm).

Radiation Doubling Dose

It is the amount of radiation a population requires to produce in the next generation as many additional mutations as arise spontaneously. It measures the risk from genetic exposure. In humans, the genetic doubling dose that results in death is approximately 2 Sv.

Radiation effects during lifetime may be immediate or delayed.

Immediate Effects

Skin: Excessive exposure to X-rays will cause erythema, dryness and desquamation of the skin. Sometimes it causes dermatitis and cracking of the skin.

Nails: They become fissured and cracked. At times, they may fully crumble down.

**Caution to the Dentist

Not to hold the film in the patient's mouth during exposure, because working constantly in the moist area and continuous washing of the hands, makes the dentist more prone to dermatitis which may lead to ulceration (Fig. 2.4).

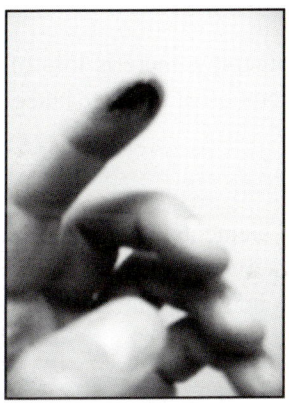

Fig. 2.4: Ulceration on the dentist's finger due to radiation exposure.

Hair: Exposure to radiation results in loss of hair called epilation. It may or may not be associated with dermatitis.

Blood forming tissue: Bone marrow and lymph nodes are susceptible to radiation and these may get damaged, leading to change in the peripheral blood count, mostly leucopenia.

Eyes: Therapeutic dosage may result in cataract formation. Still higher dosages can cause detached retina.

Lymphoid tissue: Amount of scattered radiation received by the neck is very large during dental radiographs. Lymph nodes may be affected. Therefore, the neck should be protected with a lead collar.

Reproductive organs: Irradiation of reproductive organs can give rise to sterility, but the radiation dose to the gonads is negligible with dental radiographs.

Effects on the Oral Cavity

Blood Vessels and Capillaries

Radiation causes damage to the endothelial cells in the form of degeneration and necrosis. This may cause a decrease in the lumen size. It also gives rise to peri vascular fibrosis which further narrows down the lumen.

Mucous Membrane and Epithelium

Within two weeks of the X-ray treatment, the patient develops a very agonizing condition called 'radiation mucositis', which shows erythema, ulceration, desquamation and secondary candidiasis involving the oral epithelium as a result of which, the patient has difficulty in eating and swallowing.

Taste Buds

In 2–3 weeks after radiotherapy, there is loss of taste sensation which is due to atrophy and degeneration of the taste buds. Recovery may take place after 2–3 months.

Salivary Glands

Atrophy of the glandular elements gives rise to xerostomia, i.e. decreased salivary flow and increased viscosity of the saliva. This is a predisposing factor for radiation caries and recurrent desquamation of the oral mucosa.

Periodontal Ligament (PDL)

Radiation exposure can cause disorganization of PDL fibres, decreased vascularity and increased chances of infection.

Pulp

Due to decreased vascularity and decreased cellularity, the teeth become prone to infection.

Developing Teeth

Absence of tooth, hypoplastic tooth, and decreased size of tooth are some of the effects due to damage from radiation.

Fully Developed Teeth

One of the effects of radiation on fully developed teeth is a condition called radiation caries. More than one tooth in the same region is affected. Three manifestations of radiation caries are seen. They are:

(i) Rapidly spreading caries along the neck of the teeth causing amputation of the crown.

(ii) Black discoloration of the entire surface of the tooth.

(iii) En masse destruction of the crown.

Dental caries	Radiation caries
Present mostly on the occlusal or proximal surface.	Present at the cemento – enamel junction.
Appears as a diffuse radiolucency on the radiograph.	Appears as a punched out radio-lucency seen on the radiograph (*Apple core appearance*).
Can be arrested by excavation and dressing.	Cannot be arrested.

Causes of radiation caries

(i) Xerostomia.

(ii) Lack of cleansing effect of saliva which causes food accumulation.

(iii) Absence of salivary anti-bacterial agents.

(iv) Absence of buffering action of saliva. The pH of saliva reduces, thus making it more acidic.

Treatment of radiation caries

(a) Artificial saliva can be prescribed to the patient to provide symptomatic relief from dryness. Commonly available brands in the market are *Wet mouth, Oralube.*

(b) Frequent irrigation of the mouth and sipping of water can also help treat dryness of the mouth.

(c) Fluoride containing mouth rinses (*S Flow*) can be advised to provide protection against radiation caries.

(d) Topical application of 1% Sodium fluoride gel in specially made soft plastic trays is also helpful to provide protection against caries.

(e) Dietary counseling and reduction of intake of sucrose containing food.

(f) While treating teeth affected by radiation caries endodontics is preferred to extraction in order to avoid the complication of developing osteoradionecrosis in the irradiated bone.

(g) Lactoperoxidase: Biotin toothpaste and biotin mouthwash which contain lactoperoxidase can be prescribed to the patient to counteract the effects of postradiation xerostomia.

Delayed Effects

Carcinoma

Repeated exposures to X-rays in the past are known to have caused malignancies. (Dr. Kells an early radiologist suffered from carcinoma of the upper extremity.) Patients receiving radiotherapy for treatment of malignancies can also develop secondary malignancies due to exposure to high doses of radiation. Leukemia is a more common malignancy amongst radiologists and in victims who have survived atomic explosions.

Osteoradionecrosis

It is a complication arising as a result of exposure to high doses of therapeutic radiation. As a result of high dose of radiation, the bone becomes:

(i) Hypovascular because of endothelial changes and subsequent perivascular fibrosis.

(ii) Hypoxic: As the blood does not reach the bone, oxygen supply is depleted.

(iii) Hypocellular: Ionizing radiation causes death of rapidly multiplying osteoblasts giving rise to hypocellularity.

(iv) Hypomineralised: As the bone is hypocellular with less blood supply, less mineralization takes place.

This bone becomes more susceptible to infection or trauma as vascular changes within the bone affect the defence mechanism adversely and thus trauma, infection and irradiated bone form a dangerous triad which gives rise to osteoradionecrosis.

In osteoradionecrosis, when the irradiated bone is exposed to trauma such as tooth extraction, large sequestra are formed, and the dead bone gets exposed to the oral cavity causing intense pain. Very often it gives rise to suppuration and pathological fractures. *It can be differentiated from osteomyelitis by the fact that it does not show any periosteal reaction.* (Since osteoblasts are dead or non-functioning.)

Management of Osteoradionecrosis

1. **Prevention:** It is better to prevent the occurrence of osteoradionecrosis than to cure it. Before beginning with radiotherapy of the orofacial region, a dentist should be consulted. All the carious

teeth infected root pieces and other teeth which are likely to get infected are treated before radiotherapy.

2. Avoid trauma to the irradiated bone.

3. Meticulous oral hygiene procedures to avoid caries, food impaction, infection, etc.

4. Endodontics is better than exodontia at least for two years after the radiotherapy.

5. Use of intra- or extraoral lead shield to protect the alveolar bone during radiotherapy can help to reduce the radiation dose to the bone.

6. If osteoradionecrosis occurs, antibiotics must be given to control the infection.

7. The sequestrum may be surgically removed carefully. Some investigators advocate that the sequestrum should exfoliate on its own.

8. Hyperbaric oxygen is used to prevent and control anaerobic infections and promote angiogenesis. The recommended regimen is one dive of 100% oxygen at 2.5 atmospheric pressure for 90 minutes. Many such dives are planned for the patient depending upon the severity of the case.

RADIATION PROTECTION

Radiation protection can be classified into:

1. General protection
2. Protection of patient
3. Protection of operator

General Protection

Principle of ALARA should be followed. Radiation exposure should be (*As Low As Reasonably Achievable*).

1. Restrict the number of radiographs by choosing the most appropriate views required for a particular case.

2. The chosen technique should be properly executed and repetitions must be avoided. Long cone technique helps to reduce patient exposure (Fig. 2.5).

3. Adequate filtration must be used which cuts off the long wave photons that are not diagnostically useful.

4. Adequate collimation must be used to restrict the size and the shape of the X-ray beam.

5. Use optimum kVp (A low kVp causes more radiation hazards because most of the X-rays are absorbed by the patient before reaching the film).
6. Reduce the exposure time by using fast speed films and intensifying screens.
7. Periodic maintenance of the X-ray machine to check for leakage is recommended.
8. Good processing techniques must be used to obtain good quality radiographs which will help to avoid repeating the exposure.

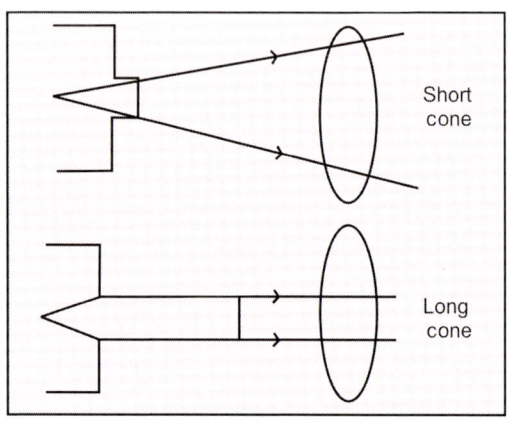

Fig. 2.5: Reduced patient exposure with long cone technique.

Protection of the Patient

1. Reduce the number of X-ray exposures.
2. Filtration, collimation and optimum kVp during exposure also contribute to reduction in patient exposure.
3. Patient exposure can be reduced by using high speed double emulsion film and intensifying screens.
4. Use of film holder to position the film can also help to reduce the patient exposure.
5. Lead apron (about 2 mm thick lead) can be used to drape the patient during exposure. Special care must be taken in case of pregnant ladies.
6. Lead goggles and lead collars can be used to protect the thyroid gland and cervical lymph nodes.
7. Ideally, the patient should maintain a record of X-ray exposure.

Protection of the Operator

1. The dentists are instructed not to hold the film in the patient's mouth. Repeated exposure of the dentist's wet fingers to radiation can lead to hazardous consequences.

2. The dentist must not stand in the direction of the central ray, i.e. always stand behind the X-ray tube. The *position-distance rule* must be followed for personal safety. According to this rule, the dentist must stand at a distance of at least 6 feet from the machine at an angle of 90–135° to the primary beam.

3. Use of a lead barrier or partition between the dentist and the X-ray machine is desirable while making the exposure.

4. While screening, a lead apron must be worn.

5. Filtration, collimation and suitable kVp must be used during every exposure.

6. The dentist must work in a well ventilated room.

7. Periodic WBC counts are advisable for the occupationally exposed.

8. Monitoring: It is a periodic and continuous determination of radiation dose in an area (area monitoring) or received by a person (personal monitoring). Personal monitors are of 3 types:
    – Pocket dosimeter
    – Film badge
    – Thermoluminescent dosimeter.

Pocket Dosimeter

It has a quartz fiber mounted on a horseshoe-shaped bar and the complete assembly is mounted in the sensitive chamber of the dosimeter. When it is exposed to X-rays, the quartz fiber loses its positive charge and starts moving away from the zero position hence direct reading can be taken.

Film Badge

A dental film is placed in a film badge having a number of windows. These windows have different metallic filters (Figs 2.6 and 2.7). At the end of two months, the film is sent to a Radiation Protection Service where it is developed and depending upon the density, the radiation exposure is calculated.

Advantage

Different types of radiation energies can be recorded using a film badge.

Disadvantage

The accuracy is only 10 to 50%.

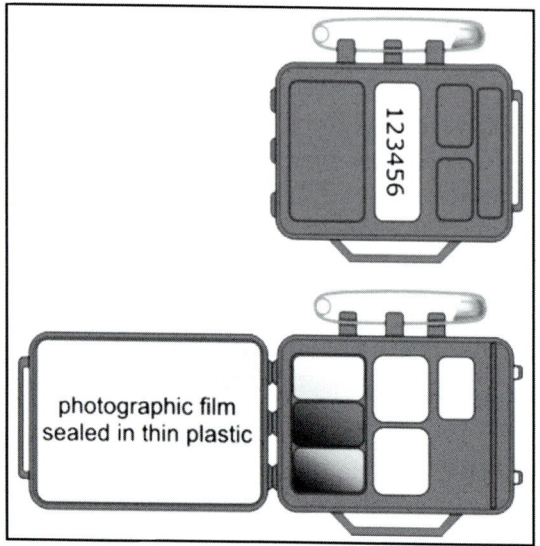

photographic film
sealed in thin plastic

123456

Fig. 2.6: Diagram of a film badge.

Cu$_1$	Cd	Open
Cu$_2$	Pb	Plastic

Fig. 2.7: Diagrammatic representation of the composition of a film badge.

Thermoluminescent Dosimeter (Figs 2.8 and 2.9)

In this dosimeter, crystalline substances like lithium fluoride or calcium sulphate diphosphor is used. These crystals undergo ionic changes when exposed to X-rays and subsequently when the crystals are heated in a special container they give out visible light which is measured by a photo-multiplier device, giving a direct reading of the exposure. Because the crystals give out visible light after heating, they are called as thermoluminescent crystals. The amount of light given out is measured which is proportional to the radiation exposure received.

Advantages

  (i) A wide range of exposures are detected.
 (ii) Accuracy is up to 30%.
(iii) Response is almost similar to human tissues.
(iv) Direct reading available at any time.
 (v) Response is independent of radiation energy.
(vi) It can be incorporated in jewelry.
(vii) Lithium fluoride crystals can be re-used.

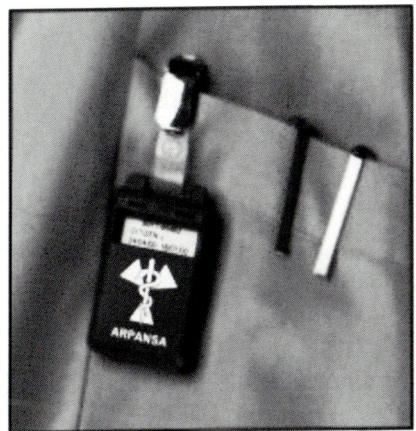

Fig. 2.8: Thermoluminescent dosimeter (TLD).

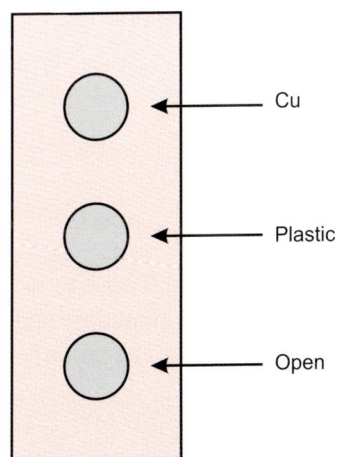

Fig. 2.9: Diagrammatic representation of the composition of a thermoluminescent dosimeter (TLD).

DOSIMETRY

ROENTGEN

Roentgen is the unit of exposure. It is that amount of X, or gamma, radiation such that the associated corpuscular emission, per 0.001293 gram of air, produces in air ions carrying 1 electrostatic unit of charge of either signs.

1 Roentgen (R) = 2.58×10^{-4} C/kg of air

The SI unit of exposure is kerma, i.e. kinetic energy released in matter. It measures the kinetic energy transferred from photons to electrons.

RADIATION ABSORBED DOSE

This is the measure of the energy absorbed from the radiation beam per unit mass of tissue. The SI unit is Gray (Gy) and measured in terms of joules/kg.

The original unit was rad which was measured in terms of ergs/gram.
1 Gray = 100 rads
1 Gray = 100 centigray

RADIATION EQUIVALENT DOSE

This is a measure that allows the different radiobiological effectiveness of different radiation types to be taken into account.

Radiation equivalent dose = rad × quality factor (Q).

The quality factor is different for different types of radiation.

For X-rays, Q = 1, for α rays, Q = 20.

The unit of radiation equivalent dose is Sievert (Sv). The traditional unit is rem (roentgen equivalent man).

1 Sv = 100 rem

For diagnostic X-rays, 1 Sv = 1 Gy.

RADIATION EFFECTIVE DOSE

It is the measure of the risk of human tissues to radiation induced damage and calculated as the product of equivalent dose and tissue weighting factor which is different for different tissues. The unit of effective dose is Sievert.

RADIOACTIVITY

Radioactivity indicates the rate of decay of a radioactive material. The SI unit is becquerel (Bq).

1 Bq = 1 disintegration/second

The traditional unit is Curie (Ci) and corresponds to the radioactivity of 1 gram of radium.

1 Ci = 3.7×10^{10} disintegrations/second

In order to monitor radiation safety, the International Commission on Radiological Protection (ICRP) has set the maximum permissible annual exposure limits for radiation workers and general public. As per its rules:

(i) Classified radiation workers are those who receive high radiation exposure at work and require compulsory personal monitoring and annual health checks. The maximum permissible annual dose to this group is 20 mSv.

(ii) Non-classified radiation workers are those who receive low levels of radiation exposure at work. Most dental staff fall into this category and the maximum permissible dose to this group is 6 mSv.

(iii) General public refers to any group which is not receiving radiation as a patient or worker, but may be inadvertently exposed to radiation. This group includes people in the waiting rooms, passers-by, etc. and the maximum permissible radiation dose is 1 mSv.

SUGGESTED READING AND REFERENCES

1. Oral Radiology: Principles and Interpretation, White and Pharoah; 5th edition.
2. Essentials of Dental Radiography and Radiology, Eric Whaites, 3rd edition.
3. Fundamental Physics of Radiology, Meredith, Massey.

Notes

CHAPTER 3

Ideal Radiograph and Radiographic Techniques

AN IDEAL RADIOGRAPH

An ideal radiograph has been defined by *H.M.Worth as the one which has the desired density or overall darkness and which shows the part completely, without distortion, with maximum detail and with the right amount of contrast to make the detail fully apparent.*

According to Wuherman, the image should be sharp and of the size and shape of the object. Radiography is nothing but a shadow casting procedure and it follows the rules of projection geometry which are as follows:

1. The source of radiation must be as small as possible.
2. The tube object distance must be as large as possible.
3. The object film distance should be as small as possible.
4. The object and film should be parallel to each other.
5. The central ray must be perpendicular to the long axis of the film and the object.

Explanation

1. If the source of radiation is large, then from each point of source a ray will emerge casting shadow at different spots. In other words one point in the object will be represented by a number of points on the image thereby making the image unsharp. This area of unsharpness is called as penumbra. Ideally a point source will cast a sharpest image, but practically it is not possible to have a point source. Hence, the line focus principle is followed. A simple example to illustrate this is that our shadow under the bulb is sharper than under the tube light which acts as a larger source (Fig. 3.1).

2. If the source of radiation is brought closer to the object, because of the divergence of the beam, the shadow is magnified and the

area of unsharpness also increases. Hence the object source distance must be as large as possible (Fig. 3.2).

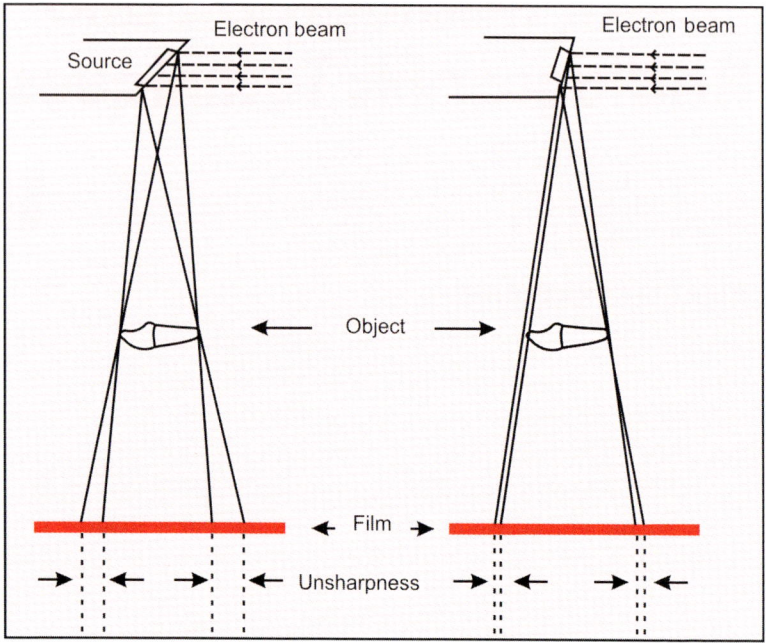

Fig. 3.1: Importance of small focal spot size.

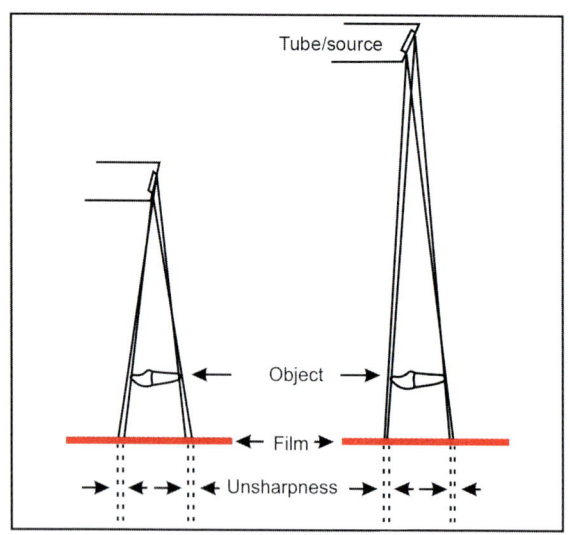

Fig. 3.2: Importance of large tube object distance.

3. If the object is placed away from the film the rays emerging from the object will be diverging giving rise to magnification and unsharpness of the image (Fig. 3.3).

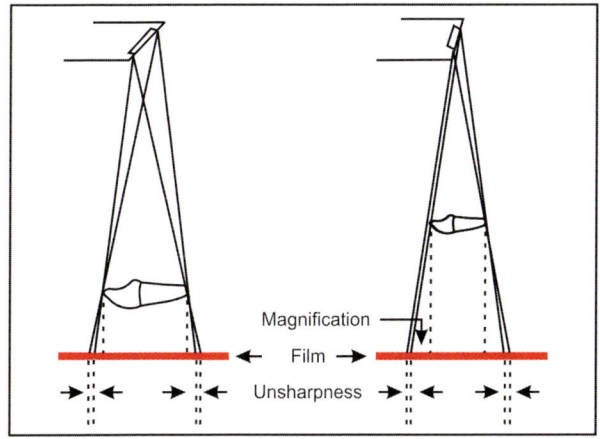

Fig. 3.3: Importance of small object film distance.

To illustrate the above two points, if you go close to the candle kept on the table, your shadow on the wall will appear magnified and unsharp, whereas if you move closer to the wall, the shadow on the wall appears sharp.

4. If the object is not parallel to the film, the size of the object is not equal to the size of the image on the film. Hence, the object and the film should be kept parallel to each other (Fig. 3.4).

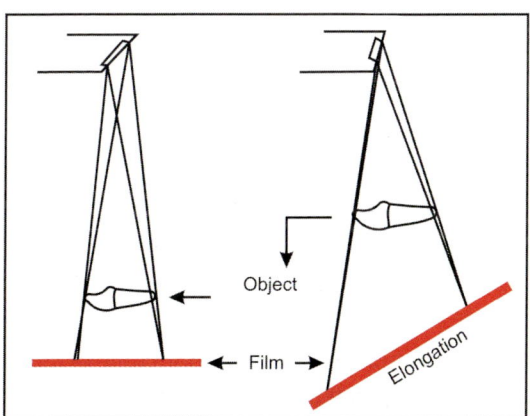

Fig. 3.4: Importance of placing object and film parallel to each other.

5. If the central ray is not perpendicular to the object/film, it will result in distortion of the image, e.g. if the central ray is perpendicular to the tooth but not the film, it will result in elongation (Fig. 3.5) and if the ray is perpendicular to the film but not to the tooth, it will result in shortening (Fig. 3.4).

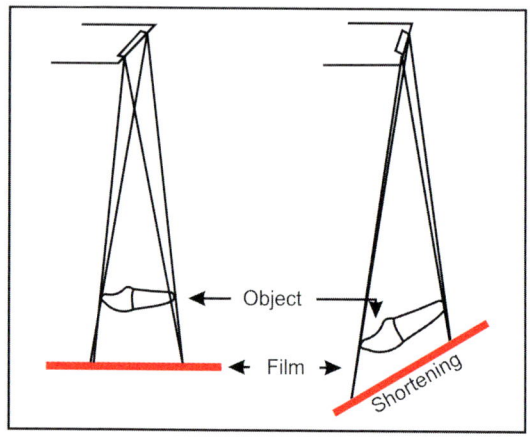

Fig. 3.5: Importance of having the central ray perpendicular to the tooth and film.

PRINCIPLE OF BISECTING ANGLE TECHNIQUE

The principle of bisecting angle technique was given by Saterlee. In this technique, the film makes an angle with the tooth since it invariably touches the incisal edge and is away from the roots. The central ray is directed at right angles to the imaginary line which bisects the angle formed by the long axis of the tooth and the long axis of the film. The target film distance is 6–8 inches.

This technique follows the *Ciezensky's rule of isometry* (Fig. 3.6b) which says that if two angles and one side of two triangles are equal then the two triangles are congruent. As a result of this, the image size becomes equal to the tooth size (Fig. 3.6a).

Effect of Improper Vertical Angulation on the Image

Excessive vertical angulation will result in shortening of the image (Fig.3.7), while less vertical angulation will result in elongation (Fig. 3.8).

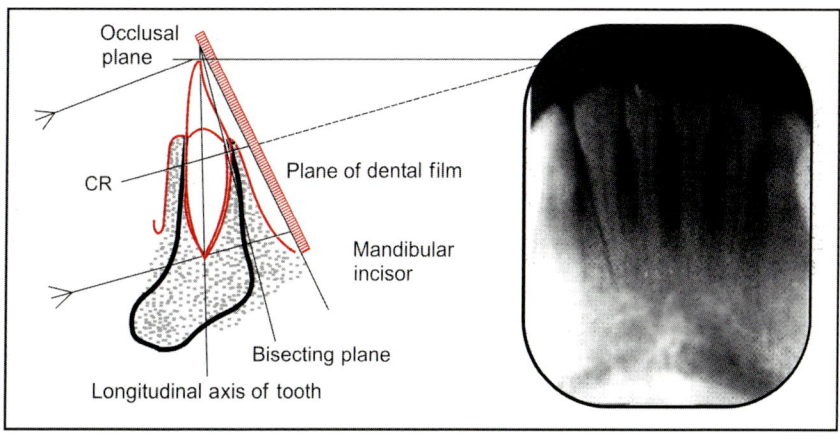

Fig. 3.6a: Principle and method of bisecting angle technique.

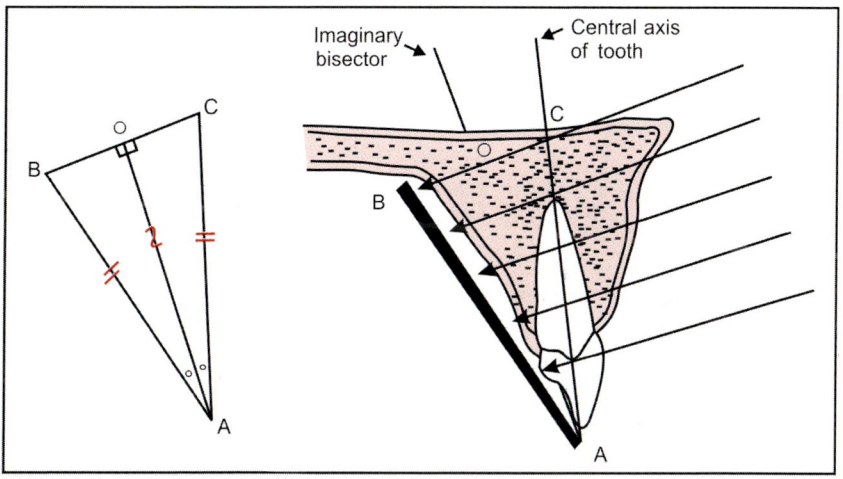

Fig. 3.6b: Diagram explaining the Ciezensky's rule of isometry.

PRINCIPLE OF PARALLELING TECHNIQUE

In this technique, a special device called the UpDegrave's device or a Rinn XCP film holder is used to position the film parallel to the tooth. The central ray is directed at right angles to the long axis of the tooth (Fig. 3.9). The target film distance for paralleling technique is 16–18 inches.

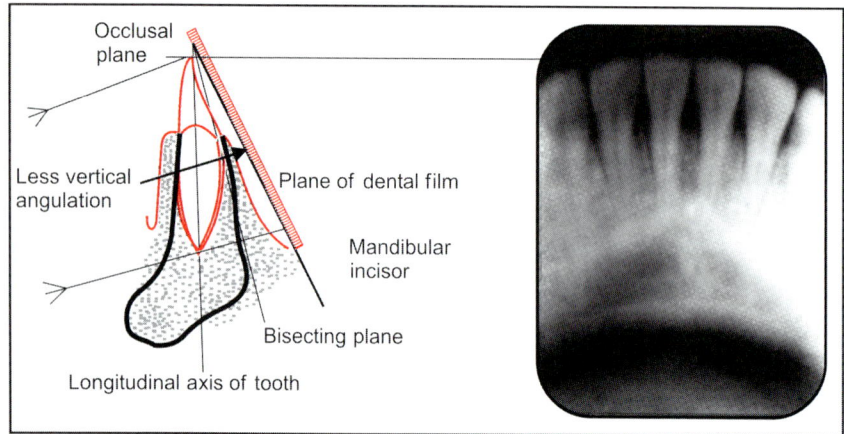

Fig. 3.7: Shortening of the image due to excessive vertical angulation.

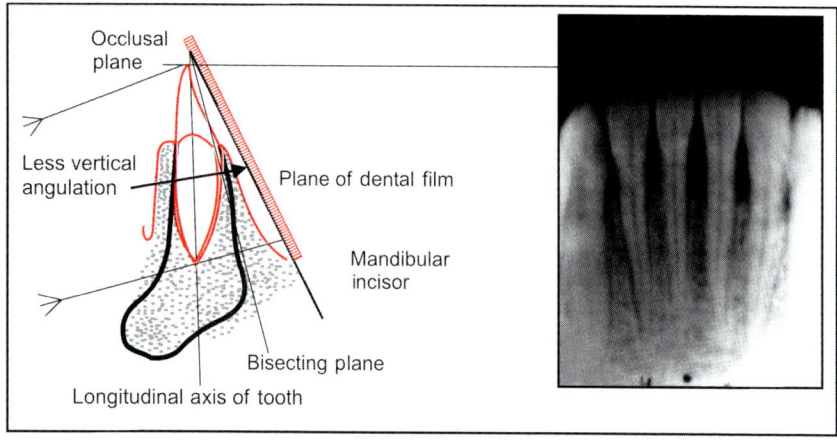

Fig. 3.8: Elongation of the image due to less vertical angulation.

CHARACTERISTICS OF RADIOGRAPHS OBTAINED WITH PARALLELING TECHNIQUE

The main difference between bisecting angle technique and paralleling technique is that in bisecting angle technique, the X-rays pass obliquely through the teeth under study thereby causing separation of the buccal and the lingual cusps and the alveolar crests. In paralleling technique, the rays pass at right angles to the tooth thereby ensuring a true lateral image of the tooth in question, i.e. the buccal and lingual cusps and the alveolar crests will exactly superimpose. In other words, the buccal and lingual crestal levels are well represented.

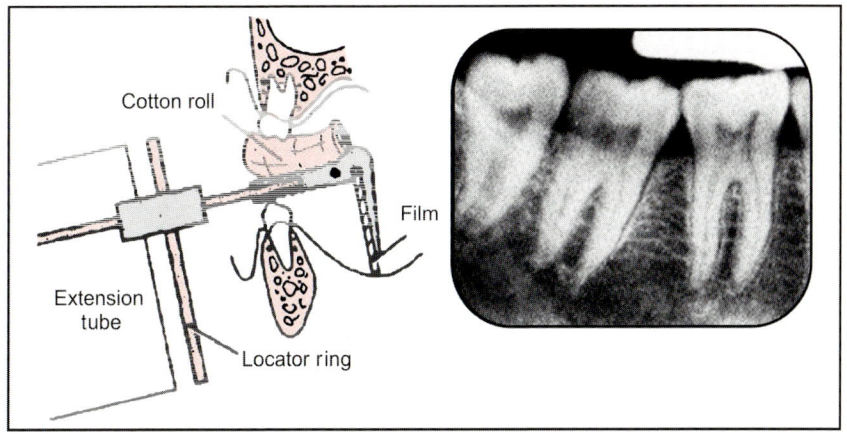

Fig. 3.9: Principle and method of paralleling technique.

Advantages of Paralleling Technique

1. There is maximum superimposition of the buccal and lingual cusps.
2. There is maximum superimposition of the buccal and lingual alveolar crests.
3. There is maximum superimposition of proximal surfaces.
4. No superimposition of zygomatic process of the maxilla on the root apices of the teeth.
5. Since the TFD is more, the X-rays are more parallel to each other and therefore there is minimum magnification and maximum sharpness and details in the image.
6. Since the rays are passing at right angles to the object and film, there is minimum foreshortening of the buccal roots of upper molars.

In bisecting angle technique, the rays are passing obliquely through the tooth and this causes foreshortening of the buccal roots.

Disadvantages of Paralleling Technique

1. Since the TFD is more, the exposure time and kVp have to be increased.
2. A film holder is required (Fig. 3.10).
3. It is a time consuming method.
4. Since the film is placed away from the tooth, there are chances of penumbra formation and magnification.
5. In cases with a shallow palate, if the film is held parallel to the tooth, the apex of the tooth might be cut off.

6. It is difficult to place the film parallel to the tooth with the rubber dam secured in position.

7. Film holding devices will have to be sterilized/disinfected to prevent cross contamination.

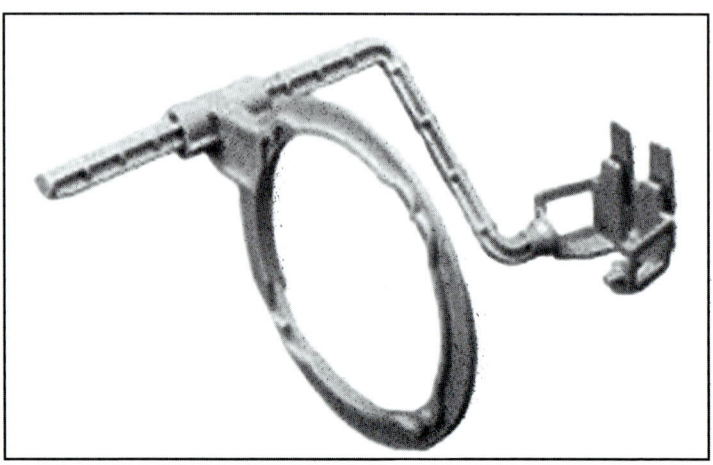

Fig. 3.10: Film holding device used in paralleling technique.

DIFFERENCES BETWEEN PARALLELING AND BISECTING ANGLE TECHNIQUE

	Bisecting angle technique	Paralleling technique
Source of radiation	Common to both	Common to both
Target film distance (Fig.3.11)	6–8 inches. The rays are more divergent and hence can cause magnification and unsharpness.	16–18 inches. The rays are nearly parallel and hence there are fewer chances of magnification and distortion.
Object film distance	The film touches the tooth and hence there is less chance of distortion.	The film is placed away from the tooth and hence there are chances of image distortion.
Position of object and film	The film is at an angle to the tooth (Fig.3.6).	The film and tooth are parallel to each other (Fig.3.9).
Central ray	The central ray is angulated so that it is perpendicular to the angle bisector	The central ray is perpendicular to the film and the object

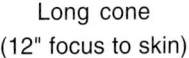

Short cone
(8" focus to skin)

Long cone
(12" focus to skin)

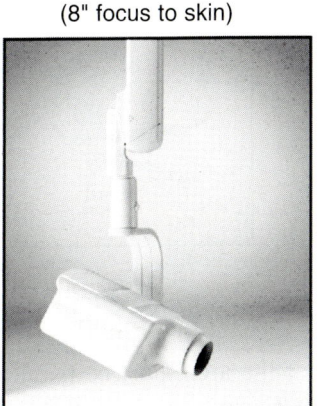
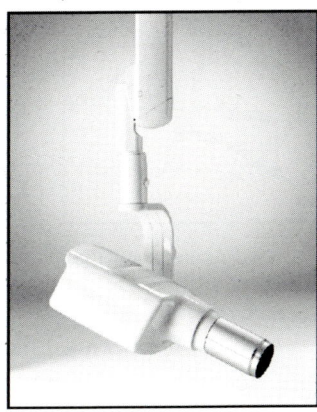

Fig. 3.11: Tube heads for short and long cone techniques.

PERIAPICAL RADIOGRAPHS

The main objective of periapical radiographs is to study the entire tooth from the incisal edge to the apex with specific stress on the periapical area.

Indications

1. To study periapical cyst, abscess and granulomas.
2. To study tooth fractures.
3. To study caries and pulpal diseases.
4. To study periodontal bone loss.
5. To study developmental defects such as dens in dente, dilacerations concrescence.
6. To study the root canal system and anatomy during endodontic treatment.
7. Implant imaging, before and after placement.

Technique

1. *Head position:*
   (i) Sagittal plane must be perpendicular to the floor.
   (ii) The ala tragus line should be parallel to the floor for the upper arch (Fig. 3.12).
   (iii) The line joining the corner of the mouth to the tragus must be parallel to the floor for the lower arch (Fig. 3.13). In other

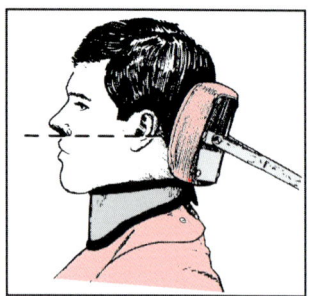

Fig. 3.12: Head position for maxillary radiographs.

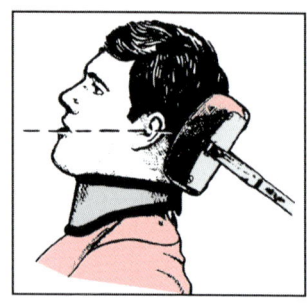

Fig. 3.13: Head position for mandibular radiographs.

words, the occlusal plane of the arch must be parallel to the floor. The patient must be instructed to remove the ornaments, spectacles or removable dentures before placing the film as these may cast a shadow on the film.

2. *Film placement:* The film is placed vertically for the anterior teeth and horizontally for the posterior teeth with the exposure side facing the tube. The tooth in question must lie at the centre of the film.

3. *Film retention:* The film is held in position by the patient himself with his thumb or index finger taking care that the fingers do not cast their shadow on the film. Film holding devices can be used to secure it in place while using the paralleling technique.

4. *TFD:*
   For bisecting angle technique   6–8 inches
   For paralleling technique   16–18 inches

5. **Centering point and vertical angulation**

Maxillary teeth		
Tooth	**Centering point**	**Angulation**
Maxillary incisors	Tip of the nose	+55°
Maxillary canines	Ala of the nose	+50°
Maxillary premolars	Meeting point of the perpendicular drawn from the mid point of the infra orbital margin to the ala tragus line.	+45°
Maxillary molars	Meeting point of perpendicular drawn from the outer canthus of the eye to the ala tragus line	+25 to +35°

Mandibular teeth		
Tooth	**Centering point**	**Angulation**
Mandibular incisors	Symphysis menti	−30°
Mandibular canines	Meeting point of the perpendicular from the ala of the nose to the lower border of the mandible.	−20°
Mandibular premolars	Meeting point of the perpendicular drawn from the mid point on the infra orbital margin to the lower border of the mandible.	−10°
Mandibular molars	Meeting point of the perpendicular drawn from the outer canthus of the eye to the lower border of the mandible.	0 to −5°

6. *Horizontal angulation:* The central ray is directed at right angles to the film through the interproximal surfaces of the teeth to be radiographed (Fig. 3.14). This can be achieved by keeping the yoke of the tube parallel to the film. Failing to use proper horizontal angulation will result in overlapping of the proximal surfaces in the resultant radiograph (Fig. 3.15).

7. Milliamperage – 10

8. kVp – 65

9. Exposure time is electronically controlled and varies from 0.4 to 0.8 second depending of the density of the region to be radiographed.

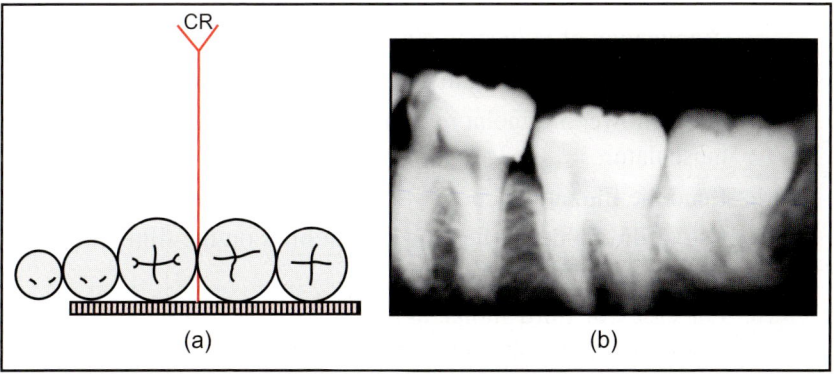

Fig. 3.14: (a) Proper horizontal angulation (b) resultant image.

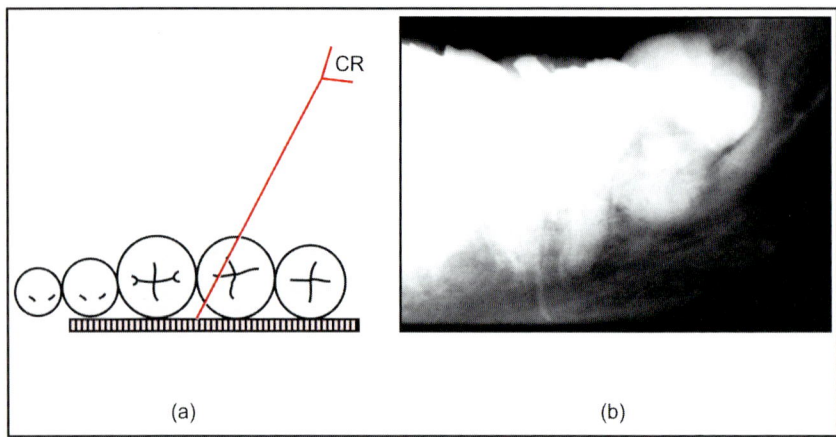

(a)   (b)

Fig. 3.15: (a) Improper horizontal angulation (b) resultant image.

METHODS TO ELIMINATE GAGGING

There are two types of stimuli that can result in gagging, the psychic and tactile stimuli. The psychic stimuli can be overcome by conditioning the patient appropriately for the radiographic examination. The tactile stimuli can be controlled by following proper techniques while film placing.

1. Keep the exposure factors and the tube placement ready before placing the film in mouth.
2. Keep the film in mouth for minimum time without sliding the film on the palate in one swift movement.
3. Divert the patient's attention by asking him to count numbers in mind.
4. Ask the patient to gargle with ice cold water.
5. Application of xylocaine ointment and spray.
6. If everything else fails, make an extra-oral radiograph.
7. For the lower 3rd molar region, ask the patient to relax his tongue musculature.
8. Bend the film at the corners so that it does not hurt.
9. Use a film holder. When the patient bites on the film holder, the floor of mouth is relaxed.
10. For cases of third molar disimpaction, the radiograph may be repeated after administering local anesthesia to the patient.

PARALLAX TECHNIQUE (CLARK'S-SLOB RULE)

This technique is used for localizing impacted teeth, foreign body, etc. in the buccolingual dimension.

While traveling in a train, a distant tree on the hill top appears to move with you, whereas an electric pole close to the railway tracks moves in the opposite direction. Similarly when two radiographs are obtained to localize an impacted tooth, if on distally moving the tube, if the tooth moves distally, it means that it is placed farther away from the tube, i.e. placed lingually. A tooth moving in the opposite direction suggest buccal placement (**S**ame **L**ingual **O**pposite **B**uccal).

METHODS TO AVOID THE SUPERIMPOSITION OF THE MALAR PROCESS ON THE ROOTS OF MAXILLARY MOLARS

1. A cotton roll can be placed between the film and the palate so that the film is moved away from the teeth. Now the vertical angulation must be reduced and the central ray is directed from below the zygomatic process of maxilla to prevent its superimposition (Fig. 3.16). This technique is called as **Le Masterís technique**.

2. The shadow of the zygomatic process of the maxilla can be shifted to study the periapical region of the tooth in question, e.g. distally tilted X-ray beam will cast a shadow of the zygoma on the periapical region of second molar, but will make the periapex of the first molar visible.

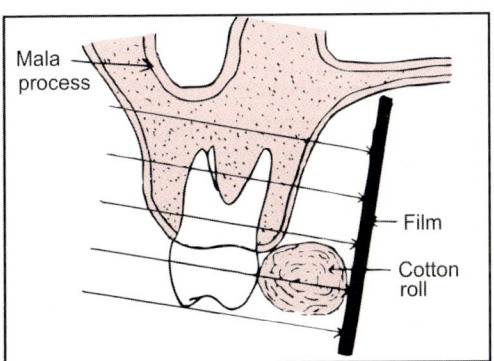

Fig. 3.16: Diagram showing the use of cotton roll to avoid the superimposition of malar process.

FAULTS/BLEMISHES/ARTIFACTS IN RADIOGRAPHS

1. *Very Light Radiograph* (Fig. 3.17)

Causes:

   (i) Underexposure
 (ii) Underdevelopment
(iii) Use of old and dilute solution
(iv) Poor quality of the film
 (v) Wrong placement of the film (lead foil towards the tube)
(vi) Decreased voltage or milliamperage

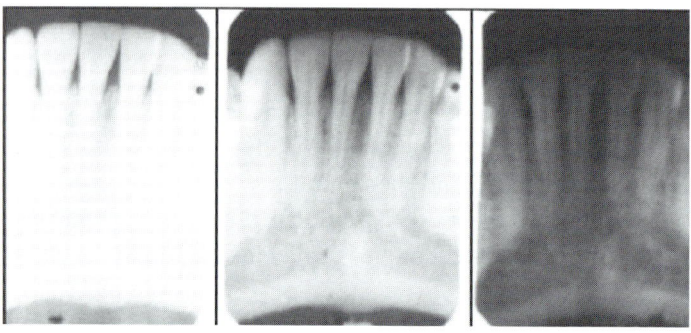

Fig. 3.17: Radiograph of a desirable density (centre), light radiograph (left), dark radiograph (right).

2. *Transparent Films*

Causes:

 (i) No exposure.

(ii) Film is put in fixer without immersing in the developer.

(iii) Spark gap (Older machines had this short circuiting device which could be activated if the voltage was too high. This would stop the generation of X-rays and protect the tube.).

3. *Very Dark Radiograph* (Fig. 3.17)

Causes:

   (i) Overexposure
 (ii) Overdevelopment
(iii) Increased temperature of developer
(iv) Accidental exposure to light

   (v) Unsafe illumination

  (vi) Increased voltage or milliamperage

Methods to make it light:

  (a) Using Farmer's solution (A and B). Farmer's solution A contains potassium ferricyanide and water, while solution B contains sodium thiosulphate and water. The two solutions are mixed and the film is immersed in it to make it light.

  (b) By scraping the emulsion from one side of the film. The developed films are immersed in the developer for some time to make the emulsion soft (effect of alkaline content). Then one side of the film is scraped to remove the emulsion completely thus making the film light.

4. *Contrast*

Excessive contrast : The film has very few areas of varying density between total white and total black.

Causes

– Low peak kilovoltage (kVp)

– Overexposure

– Overdevelopment

Insufficient contrast: The film shows multiple areas of varying density between total white and total black.

Causes

– High peak kilovoltage (kVp)

– Scattered radiation

– Underexposure

– Underdevelopment

– If intensifying screens are not used

    In order to obtain a good contrast, an optimum kVp should be used and each radiographic technique has its own optimum kVp.

5. *Blurred Radiograph*

Causes:

  (i) Large focal spot.

  (ii) Decreased TFD, therefore increased divergence of the beam.

 (iii) Movement of the patient, tube or the film (Fig. 3.18)

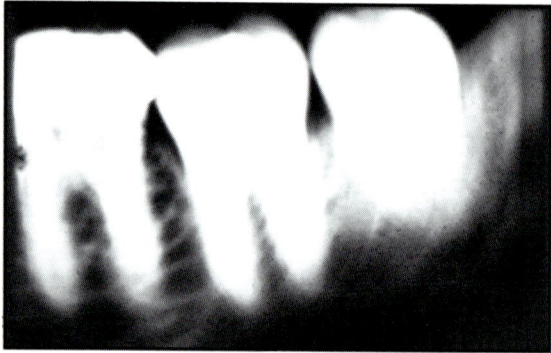

Fig. 3.18: Blurred image due to patient movement.

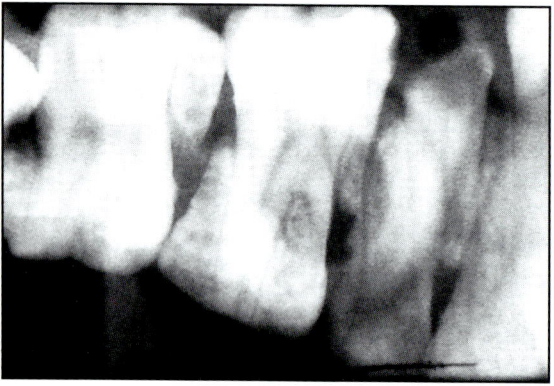

Fig. 3.19: Blurring of image due to double exposure.

(iv) Large grain size of silver bromide.

(v) Large grain size of intensifying screen crystals.

(vi) Lack of contact between the intensifying screens and the film.

(vii) Double exposure (Fig. 3.19)

6. Distorted Radiograph

The size and shape of the image is not equal to that of the object.

Causes:

(i) Excessive bending of the film.

(ii) Improper angulation of the X-ray beam.

(a) Excessive angulation causes shortening (*see* Fig. 3.7).

(b) Decreased angulation causes elongation (Fig. 3.8).

7. Fogging of the Film

Fogging is the unwanted blackening of the film caused by radiation other than the primary beam of radiation. It is of two types:

(a) General fog

Causes:

  (i) Stray radiation—exposure to light (unsafe lighting).
 (ii) Old films.
(iii) Highly oxidized developer.
 (iv) Films stored in hot and damp areas.
  (v) Frequent removal of the film from the developer and holding it against the safe light.

(b) Local fog

Causes:

  (i) Improper closure of the cassette which allows light to enter into the cassette.
 (ii) Defective wrapping of the X-ray film.

8. Stains

Yellow stains may be due to improper fixing of the film which leaves behind silver bromide crystals which when exposed to light turn yellow. They can also be due to incomplete washing of the X-ray films which leaves behind insoluble silver thiosulphate on the film.

9. White Spots

Causes:

  (i) due to the air bubbles sticking on the emulsion during developing. To avoid this one must stir the hanger during developing.
 (ii) due to fixer splash on the film before developing (Fig. 3.20).

10. Blistering/Frilling of the Emulsion

Causes:

  (i) Due to high temperature of the developer (freshly prepared developer).
 (ii) Prolonged washing of the film.
(iii) Improper rinsing.

11. Pitted Radiograph

Caused due to insufficient rinsing which gives rise to liberation of carbon dioxide gas because of acid-alkali reaction.

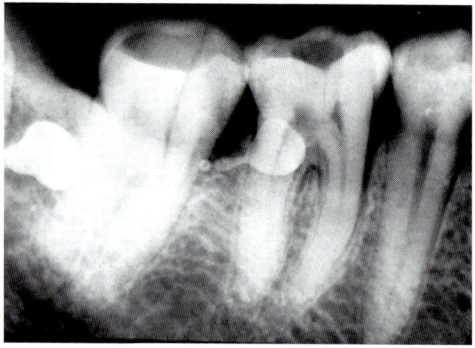

Fig. 3.20: White spots on the film due to fixer splash.

12. Kink Mark

Kink marks are caused due to abrupt or sharp bending of the film.

13. Finger Marks

If the fingers are contaminated with the developer, finger prints may be seen as a large shadow on the film.

14. Abrasion Marks

They are caused due to rough handling of the film. As a result of the abrasion, the emulsion gets scraped off giving rise to a radiopaque, linear artifact.

15. Foreign Images

– Nose rings, spectacles, ear rings, etc.
– Fingers.
– Orthodontic plates and dentures.

16. Reticulation

If the temperature of the developer is very high and that of the water or fixer is very low, the gelatin undergoes excessive swelling and sudden shrinkage, giving rise to reticulation (Fig. 3.21a).

17. Herring Bone/ Tyre-track Pattern

It is caused by the lead foil in the film packet, when the wrong side of the film is exposed to the X-rays (Fig. 3.21b).

(A) Faults while making a radiograph

   (i) Pressure marks while writing on the film.

  (ii) Wrong placement of the film.

        (a) Herring bone/tyre-track (Fig. 3.21b)

        (b) Cone cut

(iii) Bending of the film

(iv) Faulty kVp, mA and TFD.

(v) Exposure time: over/ under/ no exposure

(vi) Faulty angulation

      (a) Vertical: – Increased will cause shortening

                   – Decreased will cause elongation

      (b) Horizontal: overlapping of the proximal surfaces

(vii) Excessive salivation and light leakage

(viii) Movement unsharpness, giving rise to blurred/hazy radiograph

(ix) Double exposure (Fig. 3.18)

(x) Foreign bodies.

(B) Faults arising during processing

(i) Unsafe dark room, light leakage.

(ii) Developing faults: over/under /no development.

(iii) Fixation faults:

      (a) less fixation gives rise to stains.

      (b) Excessive fixation gives rise to light images.

(iv) Washing time:

      (a) less will cause stains.

      (b) excessive will cause swelling of the emulsion which peels off.

(v) Air bubbles

(vi) Reticulation caused by temperature difference (Fig. 3.21a).

(vii) Low level of developer causes partial image if the film is not fully immersed.

(viii) Splash of developer or fixer (Fig. 3.20).

(ix) Clip marks

(x) Contact of the film with the tank or other films during developing (Fig. 3.21c).

(xi) Fingerprints

(xii) Static electricity: during the cold season if the film is removed abruptly from the packet, static electricity is developed, which gives rise to a *naked tree-like or smudge-like pattern* which appears dark.

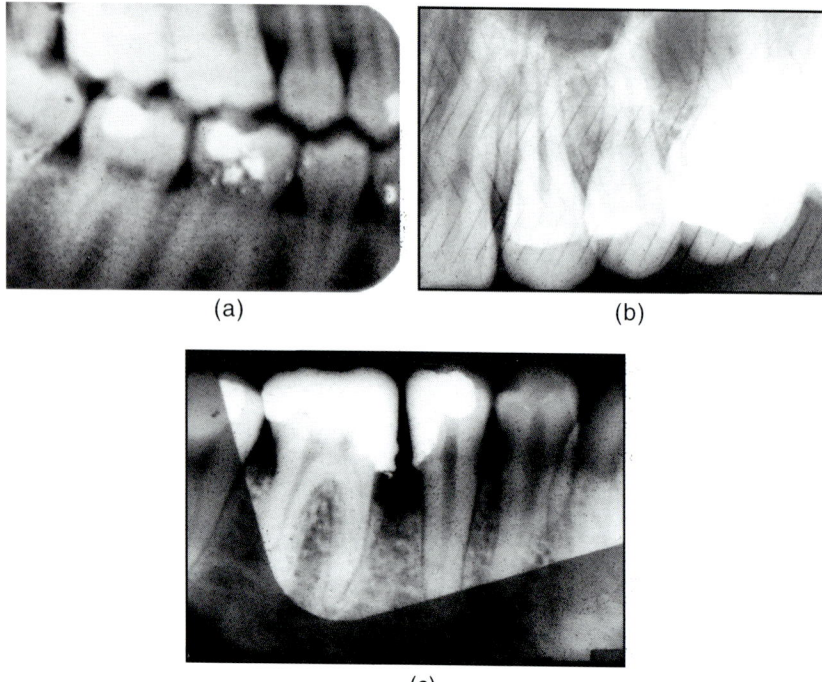

(a)

(b)

(c)

Fig. 3.21: (a) A radiograph showing reticulation,(b) A radiograph showing herring bone pattern due to reverse placement of film,(c) Artifact due to contact of film with another film during developing.

(C) Miscellaneous

(i) Scratches while handling the film.

(ii) Manufacturing defects like defects in the X-ray machines.

ANATOMICAL LANDMARKS

Tooth

Since the enamel contains 96% of mineralized component, it appears more radiopaque. Just below the enamel, dentine is seen as less radiopaque because it contains only 65% mineralized components. The pulp chamber and the root canals appear as radiolucent shadows because they contain only soft tissues. Dentine and cementum cannot be differentiated radiographically since they contain nearly the same amount of mineralized tissues.

Periodontal Ligament

The tooth is suspended in a socket by the periodontal ligament. It appears as a radiolucent thin dark line surrounding the root (Fig. 3.22). The width of this space on the radiograph is variable but usually thinnest in the mid root region. Absence of periodontal ligament space may be suggestive of ankylosis of tooth while widening is seen in conditions like apical periodontitis, scleroderma, osteosarcoma (Garrington's sign), leukemias.

Lamina Dura

It is a radiopaque line that is seen along the roots of the teeth adjacent to the periodontal ligament space (Fig. 3.22). It is the bony wall which lines the socket. As the rays have to traverse through the entire length of the structure, the lamina dura absorbs more X-rays and appears more radiopaque. The appearance of lamina dura is related to the shape of the root and consequently the shape of the bony wall of socket, e.g. mesial root of lower molars which appears dumb bell shaped in cross section presents as four separate ligament spaces and lamina dura shadows on the radiographs. Such an appearance is seen due to the configuration of the root and should not be mistaken for a fracture line.

Discontinuity of lamina dura around the roots is often a sign of disease although in certain instances, it may be thin and not discernible on the radiograph even in the absence of disease. Localised disappearance of lamina dura may be seen in periapical abscess, granuloma, etc. Generalized loss of lamina dura may be noted in hyperparathyroidism, osteoporosis, osteomalacia, etc.

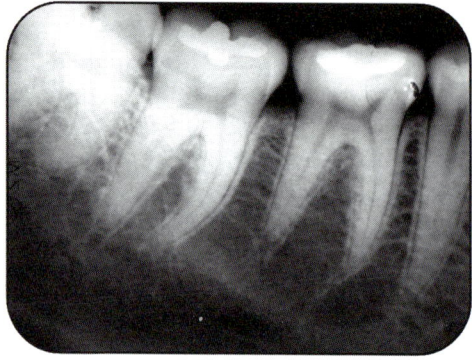

Fig. 3.22: Radiograph showing lamina dura (radiopaque) and periodontal ligament space (radiolucent) around the roots of the molars and premolar.

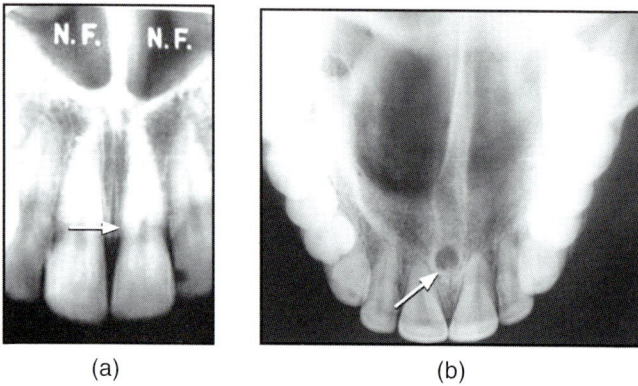

(a)   (b)

Fig. 3.23: (a) Radiograph showing the nasal fossa (NF), incisive foramen (arrow) (b) Radiograph showing the incisive foramen (arrow).

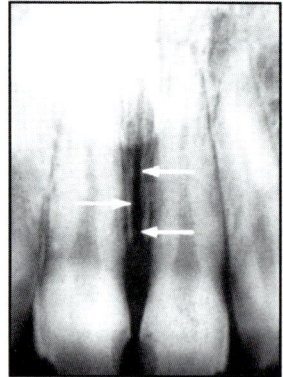

Fig. 3.24: Radiograph showing the mid palatine suture (arrows).

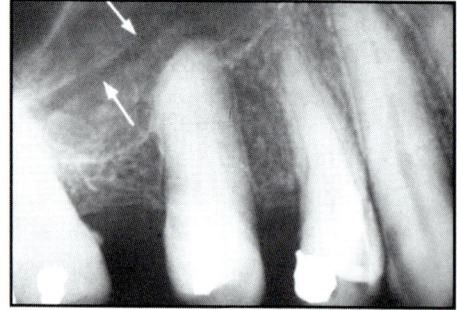

Fig. 3.25: Radiograph showing the maxillary antrum and the nutrient channels (arrows).

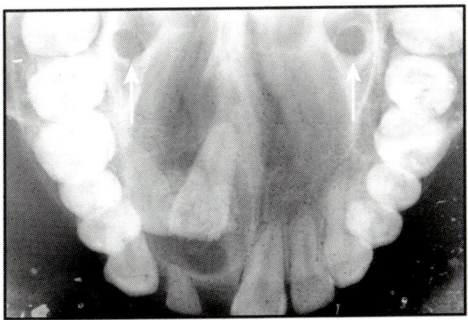

Fig. 3.26: Radiograph showing orbital opening of naso-lacrimal duct in an occlusal view (arrow).

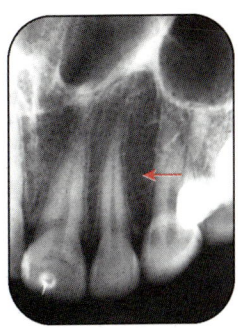

Fig. 3.27: Radiograph showing the lateral fossa (arrow).

Anatomic Landmarks of the Maxilla

Radiolucent Landmarks

1. Nasal cavity and the nasal fossa (Fig. 3.23)
2. Mid palatine suture (Fig 3.24)
3. Incisive foramen (Fig. 3.23)
4. Nostril spots (soft tissue shadow of the nose)
5. Maxillary antrum (Fig. 3.25)
6. Orbital opening of the naso-lacrimal duct (Fig. 3.26)
7. Nutrient canals—seen as grooves in the maxillary sinus (Fig. 3.25)
8. Lateral fossa (Fig. 3.27)

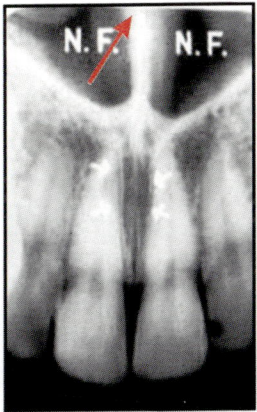

Fig. 3.28: Radiograph showing the nasal septum (arrow).

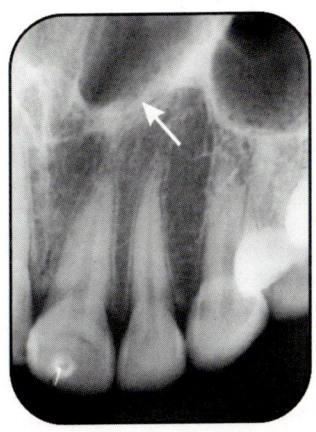

Fig. 3.29: Radiograph showing the floor of nasal cavity (arrow).

Radiopaque Landmarks

1. Nasal septum (Fig. 3.28)

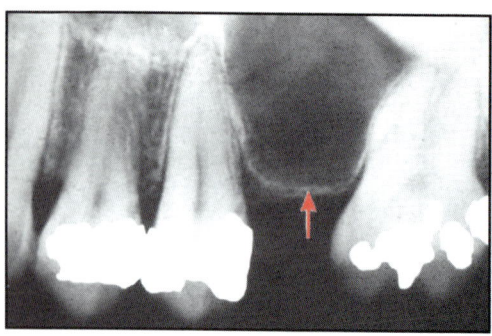

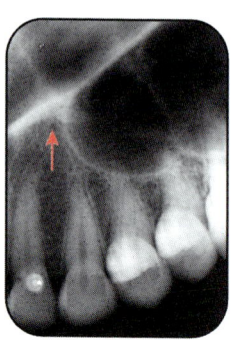

Fig. 3.30: Radiograph showing the floor of maxillary sinus (arrow).

Fig. 3.31: Radiograph showing the inverted Y line of Ennis.

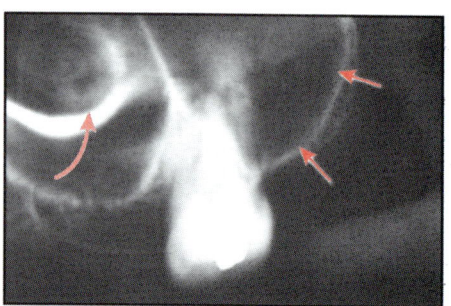

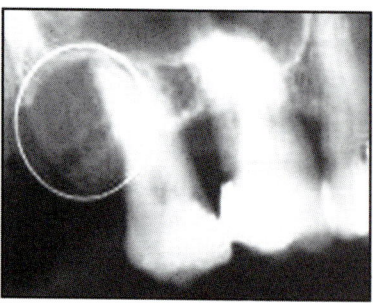

Fig. 3.32: Radiograph showing the malar process (curved arrow) and floor of maxillary sinus (red arrows).

Fig. 3.33: Radiograph showing the maxillary tuberosity.

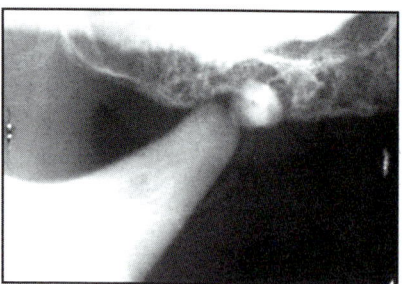

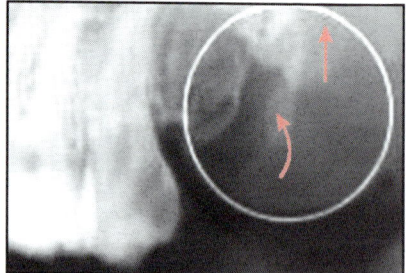

Fig. 3.34: Radiograph showing coronoid process.

Fig. 3.35: Radiograph showing pterygoid plate (straight arrow), hamular process (curved arrow).

2. Floor of the nasal cavity (Fig. 3.29)
3. Anterior nasal spine
4. Inferior nasal concha
5. Floor of the maxillary sinus (Fig. 3.30)
6. Inverted Y line of Ennis (Fig. 3.31)
7. Malar process of the maxilla (Fig. 3.32)
8. Nasolabial fold
9. Maxillary tuberosity (Fig. 3.33)
10. Coronoid process (Fig. 3. 34)
11. Pterygoid plates (Fig. 3.35)
12. Hamular process (Fig. 3.35)
13. Septum in the sinus (Fig. 3.36)

Anatomical Landmarks on the Mandible

Radiolucent Landmarks

1. Lingual foramen (Fig. 3.37)
2. Mental foramen (Fig. 3.38)
3. Mandibular foramen (seen in the ramus)
4. Mandibular canal (Fig. 3.39)
5. Submandibular gland fossa (Stafne's bone cyst) (Fig. 3.40)
6. Vascular channels (Fig. 3.40)

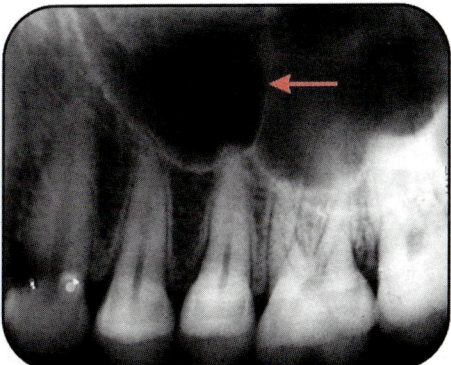

Fig. 3.36: Radiograph showing septum in the sinus (arrow).

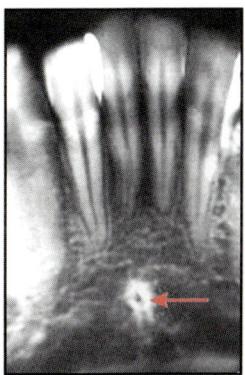

Fig. 3.37: Radiograph showing lingual foramen surrounded by genial tubercules (arrow).

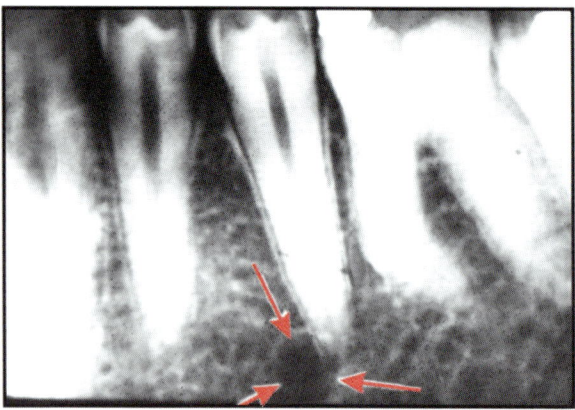

Fig. 3.38: Radiograph showing mental foramen (arrows).

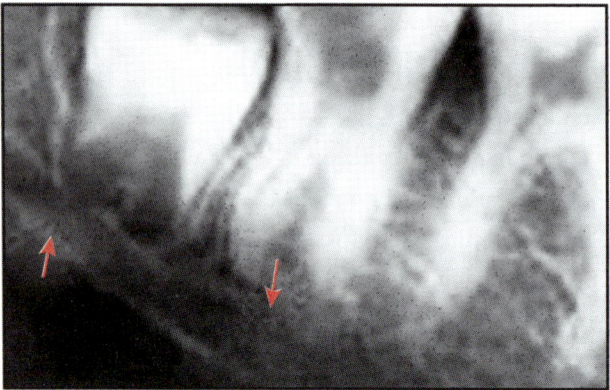

Fig. 3.39: Radiograph showing mandibular canal and tram lines (arrows).

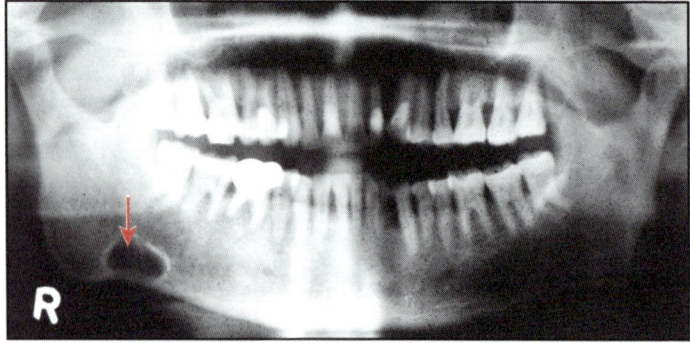

Fig. 3.40: Radiograph showing submandibular gland fossa (arrow).

7. Pharyngeal air space (seen on lateral oblique and other extra oral views)
8. Bone marrow space (Fig. 3.42)

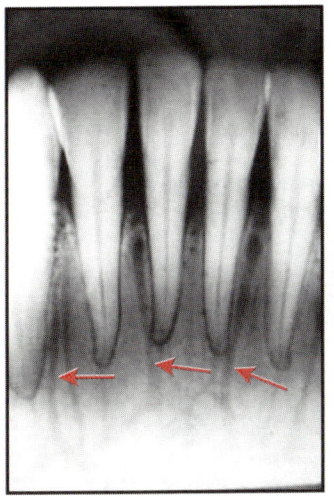

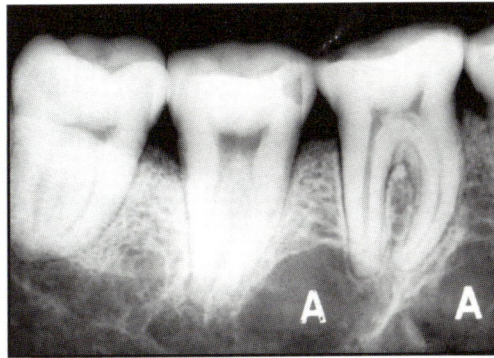

Fig. 3.41: Radiograph showing vascular channels.

Fig. 3.42: Radiograph showing large marrow spaces in the mandible (A).

Radiopaque Landmarks

1. Genial tubercles: These are seen better on true occlusal views (Fig. 3.43).
2. Mental ridge (Fig. 3.44)

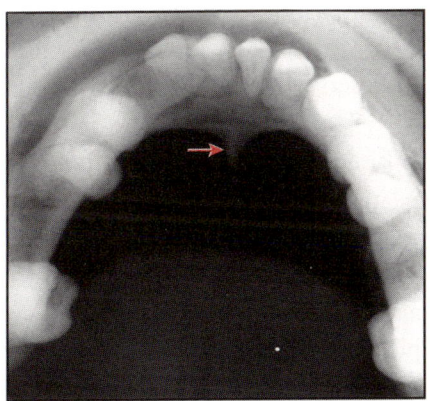

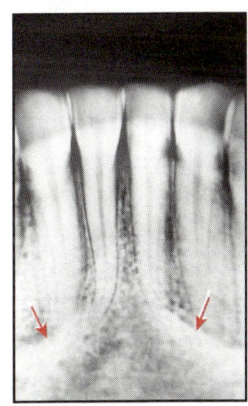

Fig. 3.43: Genial tubercles in the mandibular occlusal view (arrow).

Fig. 3.44: Mental ridge (arrows).

3. Borders of the mandibular canal (Tram lines) (Fig. 3.39)
4. External oblique ridge (Fig. 3.45)
5. Internal oblique/mylohyoid ridge (Fig. 3.45)
6. Lower border of the mandible
7. Antegonial notch
8. Condyles
9. Coronoid process
10. Sigmoid notch

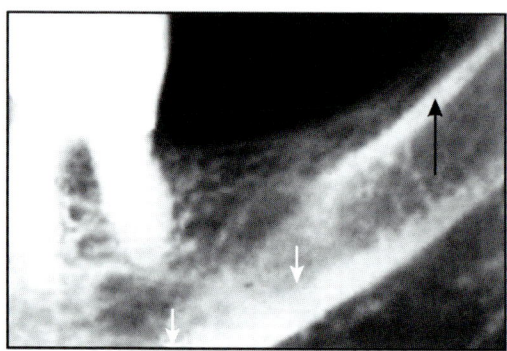

Fig. 3.45: External oblique ridge (black arrow), mylohyoid ridge (white arrows).

It should be remembered that anatomical landmarks should not be mistaken for pathologies and at the same time pathologies should not be neglected as variations of anatomical landmarks.

To differentiate between mid palatine suture (MPS) and fracture line:

(i) MPS appears like a straight line while a fracture is always a zig zag line.

(ii) Fracture has no radiopaque borders while an MPS line will usually show radiopaque borders.

To differentiate between mental foramen and periapical pathology:

(i) In case of mental foramen, the lamina dura around the root in question is intact and traceable, whereas a periapical pathology presents with discontinuous lamina dura.

(ii) By changing the horizontal angulation, the mental foramen shifts its position, while a periapical lesion will still remain attached to the tooth.

The same technique holds good to differentiate maxillary sinus and the incisive foramen from peri apical radiolucent pathologies.

BITEWING RADIOGRAPHS

INDICATIONS

1. To detect early proximal caries.
2. To study the progression of caries towards the pulp chamber.
3. To study the pulp chamber for presence of internal resorption, pulp calcifications, etc.
4. To detect early crestal bone loss.
5. To check the gingival fit of class II restorations.
6. To study the relationship of developing permanent teeth to deciduous teeth while planning for serial extractions.

TECHNIQUE

Technique of Bitewing Radiography was Given by Raper

(i) The bitewing film has a tab or a flap attached to it on which the patient bites in centric occlusion for the posterior teeth and with an edge-to-edge contact for anterior teeth (Fig. 3.46).

(ii) The central ray is directed +5° to +8° (downwards) to compensate for the curve of Monson (Fig. 3.47).

(iii) The centering point is at the occlusal plane and the central ray passes through the interproximal areas of the teeth and meets the film at right angles. Failure to use a proper horizontal angulation as mentioned above will result in proximal overlapping of the images.

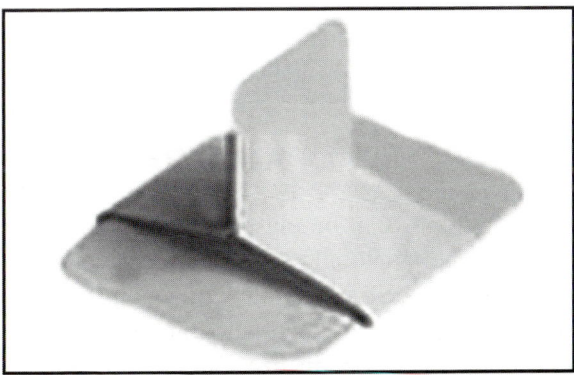

Fig. 3.46: A bitewing film.

kVp—65

mA—10

Exposure time—0.3–0.5 second

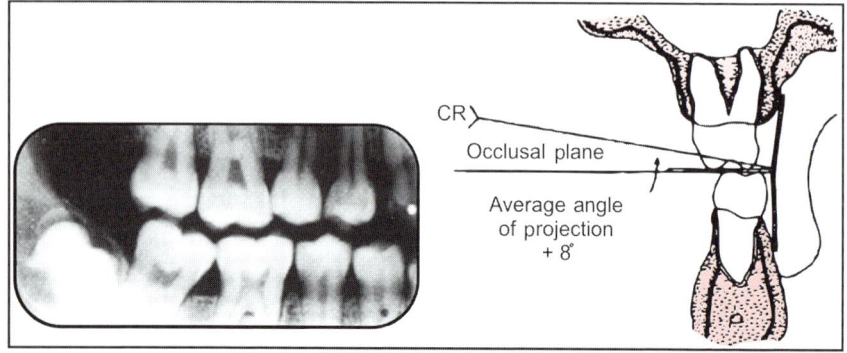

Fig. 3.47: Technique for bitewing radiographs.

Advantages of Bitewing Technique

(a) The central ray passes at right angles to film therefore there is minimum superimposition and the proximal surfaces are seen clearly. Since the rays pass obliquely in bisecting angle technique, superimposition of the tooth over tooth takes place which is not seen with bitewing radiographs.

(b) The centering point is at the level of the occlusal plane. Hence, the crown is seen well on bitewing radiographs.

(c) In a single film, the crowns of 6–8 teeth can be seen completely.

(d) Exposure to the patient is less with bitewing radiography compared to full mouth radiographs.

(e) Bitewing radiographs serve well for survey purposes.

OCCLUSAL RADIOGRAPHY

The occlusal radiographs can be classified into the maxillary and the mandibular views. The mandibular and maxillary views can be further divided into the true and the topographic views along with other modified types. The mandibular occlusal view radiograph is made with a standard occlusal film packet 57 × 76 mm in size. But for a maxillary true occlusal view, a special intraoral cassette with intensifying screen and a suitable screen film is required. The central ray is directed through the bregma and hence has to pass through the dense bones of the skull resulting in a high radiation exposure. An intraoral cassette with intensifying screens is thus used with an intention to reduce patient exposure.

True Occlusal Views (Figs 3.48 and 3.50)

Indications

1. To localize impacted, unerupted, supernumerary teeth.
2. To localize foreign bodies.
3. To study calculus in the Wharton's duct.
4. To study the buccolingual expansion of pathological processes.
5. To study displacement of fracture fragments.

Topographic Occlusal View (Figs 3.49 and 3.51)

Indications

1. To study large areas of pathological involvement which are not covered completely in intraoral radiographs.
2. To study the root length of particular teeth in an arch.
3. To detect and locate the extent of fracture line.
4. To detect impacted, unerupted, supernumerary teeth.
5. For gross examination of maxilla/mandible.
6. To study oro-antral communication, displaced root in the antrum.

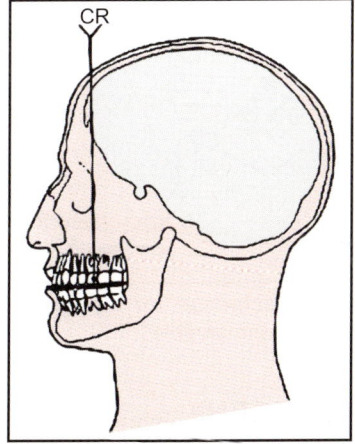

Fig. 3.48: Technique for true occlusal view of maxilla.

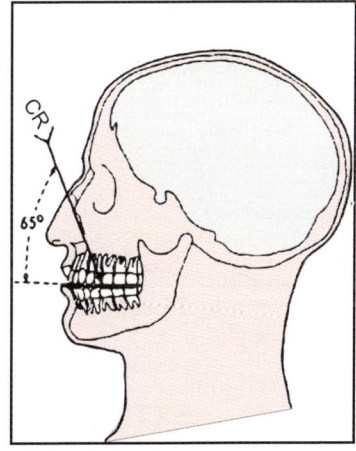

Fig. 3.49: Technique for topographic occlusal view of maxilla.

Techniques of Occlusal Radiography

	Maxillary topographic view	Mandibular topographic view	Maxillary true occlusal view	Mandibular true occlusal view
Film	57 × 76 mm Embossed dot faces the tube	57 × 76 mm Embossed dot faces the tube	57 × 76 mm screen film in a cassette	57 × 76 mm Embossed dot faces the tube
Centering point	Similar to IOPA view	Similar to IOPA view	Bregma	1/2 inch below the symphysis
Angulation	+65°	−35°	90°	90°
kVp	65	65	65	65
mA	10	10	10	10
Exposure time	0.8 sec	0.8 sec	0.8 sec	0.8 sec
TFD	30 cm	30 cm	45 cm	30 cm

To study the impacted lower third molars, the film is placed as far back as possible and the patient is asked to bite on it gently. The patient's head is tilted downwards and forwards so that the angle of mandible becomes prominent. The beam is now directed at an angle to the mandible so that the central ray is perpendicular to the film. This view gives a good picture of the impacted third molar in a bucco-lingual plane. This is called the *Donovan's technique.*

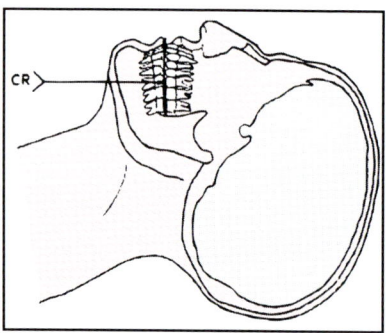 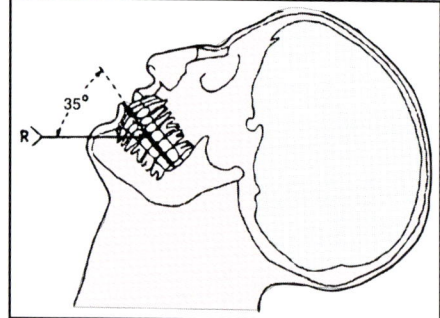

Fig. 3.50: Technique for true occlusal view of mandible.

Fig. 3.51: Technique for topographic occlusal view of mandible.

EXTRAORAL RADIOGRAPHY

Extraoral radiographs are indicated in cases where intraoral views may not provide the required information. They are particularly useful to study cases of trauma, large cysts or tumors affecting the jaws, diseases of TMJ, maxillary sinuses, etc. The following terminologies are important while describing the patient positioning for extraoral radiographs.

MID SAGITTAL OR MEDIAN PLANE (MSP)

It is a vertical plane passing through the sagittal suture between the two parietal bones. In cephalometric radiography and lateral views the sagittal plane is parallel to the cassette, while in PA views it is kept perpendicular to the cassette.

INFRAORBITAL LINE

It is a horizontal line which joins the infraorbital margins on both the sides.

CANTHOMEATAL LINE (CML) OR THE RADIOGRAPHIC BASE LINE

This is an imaginary line which joins the central point of the external auditory meatus with the outer canthus of the eye. For a PA Caldwell view, the CML is perpendicular to the cassette, while for Water's projection, CML is kept at   an angle of 45° to the cassette.

FRANKFORT HORIZONTAL PLANE (F-H plane)

 It is a plane which passes through the points Orbitale and the Porion. The Orbitale is the lowest point on the infraorbital margin, while the porion is the highest point on the external auditory meatus (Fig. 3.52).

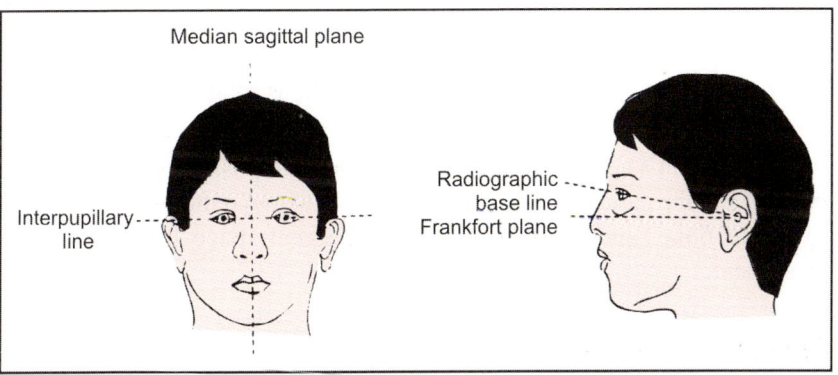

Fig. 3.52: Various reference planes for extraoral radiography.

LATERAL OBLIQUE VIEW

Indications

1. Gross examination of maxilla/mandible.
2. Examination of patients having trismus.
3. Examination of the teeth and jaws of children who cannot tolerate intraoral film.
4. To detect and locate impacted, unerupted and supernumerary teeth.
5. To detect and locate cysts, tumors and other pathologies.
6. To detect and locate fracture line.

Head Position

Since the maxilla and mandible are horseshoe-shaped bones, patient's head has to be rotated in relation to the cassette so as to study a particular area without superimposition of the opposite side. Three points to be remembered while making a lateral oblique projection are:

(i) The area to be imaged must lie in the centre of the cassette.
(ii) The area should be in close contact with the cassette.
(iii) The long axis of the teeth should be parallel with the cassette.

In order to study the various regions of the jaws, the sagittal plane has to be rotated by certain degrees of angulations. They are as follows:

(a) To study the ramus, the sagittal plane may be rotated by 10° towards the cassette.
(b) To study the molars, the sagittal plane is rotated by 15° towards the cassette.
(c) To study the premolars, the sagittal plane is rotated 30° towards the cassette and the nose tip touches the cassette.
(d) To study the canines, the sagittal plane is rotated by 45° towards the cassette.
(e) To study the incisors, the sagittal plane is rotated 60° towards the cassette and the nose is bent on the cassette.

The patient's neck is stretched to avoid superimposition of the vertebral column and the patient is asked not to swallow to avoid the superimposition of hyoid bone, and preventing the pharyngeal space from becoming prominent.

Film and Cassette

A 5 × 7 inch cassette with intensifying screens is used. There are three methods by which the cassette may be positioned:

(i) The cassette is held in hand by the patient himself.

(ii) The cassette is kept on an angle board at an angle of 23°.

(iii) The cassette may be kept flat on a table.

Centering Point

(i) For mandible, the centering point is one inch behind the angle of the mandible on the opposite side.

(ii) For the maxilla, the centering point is one inch above and behind the angle of the mandible on the opposite side.

(iii) To study the ramus, the cone may be centered below the mandibular first molar tooth of the opposite side (Fig. 3.53).

Direction of the Central Ray

The central ray passes through the radiographic key hole that is bound by the cervical spine medially and the posterior border of the mandible laterally.

Angulation: 14° upwards

TFD – 14 inches

kVp – 65, mA – 10

Exposure time – 1–1.5 second

TRUE LATERAL VIEW

Unlike the lateral oblique view, there is a complete superimposition of the right and left sides of the jaws. There are three types of true lateral views: the lateral skull view, the profile view and the cephalometric view.

Lateral Skull View

Indications

1. Facial bones
   (i) To study fractures of the nasal bone, maxilla.
   (ii) To study cysts, tumors and malignancies in the maxillary antrum.
   (iii) To study the posterior wall of maxillary sinus.
   (iv) To localize foreign bodies.
2. Cranial bones: To study changes occurring in the cranial bones such as:
   (i) Hair on end appearance in thalassemia.
   (ii) Multiple punched out radiolucencies in multiple myeloma, metastatic malignancies and eosinophilic granuloma.
   (iii) Cotton wool appearance of Paget's disease.

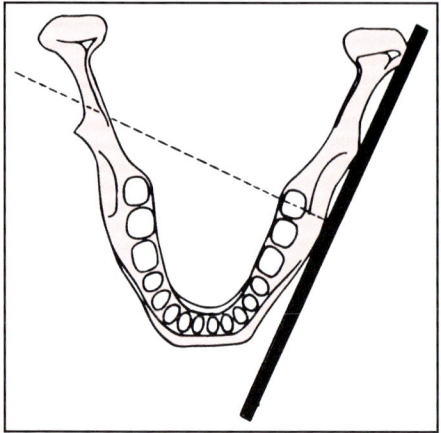

Fig. 3.53: Direction of central ray for lateral oblique view.

Head Position (Fig. 3.54)

   (i) The sagittal plane is parallel to the cassette.

  (ii) The infraorbital line is perpendicular to the cassette.

 (iii) Canthomeatal line is parallel to the floor.

 (iv) The teeth are closed in centric occlusion.

Film and Cassette

An 8 × 10 inch or 10 × 12 inch high speed film is used with suitable intensifying screens in a cassette.

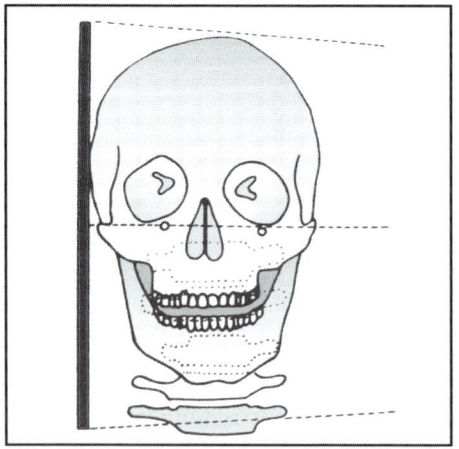

Fig. 3.54: Patient positioning for true lateral view.

Centering Point

(a) For the facial bone: The beam is centered at a point one inch below the outer canthus of the eye.

(b) For the cranial bones: The beam is centered through a point one inch in front and above the external auditory meatus.

Angulation

The central ray is directed at 90° to the cassette. The resultant radiograph is shown in Fig. 3.56.

TFD – 3 feet.

Exposure factors:

(a) Facial bones – 60 kVp, 50 mA

(b) Cranial bones – 80 kVp, 50 mA

For cephalometric view, the TFD is increased to 5 feet so as to reduce the magnification. The patient is fixed in a transmeatal axis by means of ear rods. An orbital pointer is used to indicate the orbitale. The central ray passes through the central axis of the ear rods, i.e. the external auditory meatus on both the sides (Fig. 3.55).

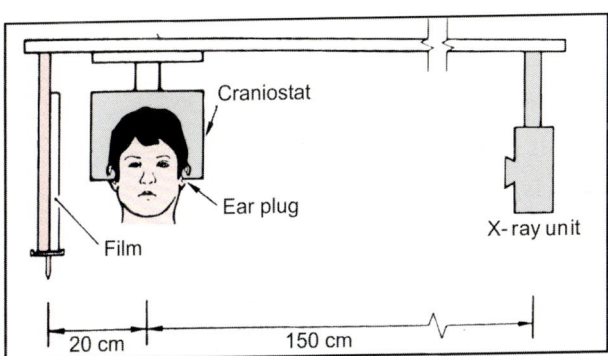

Fig. 3.55: Patient positioning for lateral cephalometry.

PA CALDWELL VIEW

Indications

1. Gross examination of the maxilla and mandible.

2. To study large lesions of the jaws like cyst, tumors.

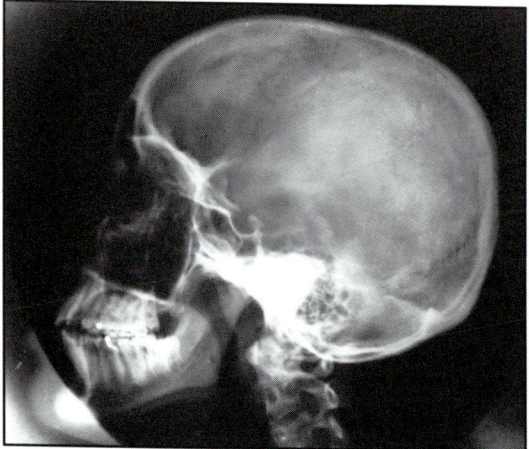

Fig. 3.56: True lateral view.

3. To study the fractures of the mandible along with displacement.
4. To study fractures of the skull bones.

In the PA Caldwell view, the entire mandible from one condyle to the other can be studied. A modification of this view in which the centering point is closer to the mandible is called as the PA mandible view. The mandible is seen more clearly in this view.

Head Position (Fig. 3.57)

(i) MSP is perpendicular to the cassette.
(ii) CML is perpendicular to the cassette.
(iii) The patient may be positioned in the forehead-nose position.

Film and Cassette

An 8 × 10 inch or 10 × 12 inch cassette is used with a suitable intensifying screen.

Centering Point

The central ray passes through a point 2 inches above the external occipital protuberance. The resultant radiograph is shown in Fig. 3.58.

Angulation – The central ray is directed at 90° to the cassette.

TFD – 3 feet

kVp – 80

mAS – 150

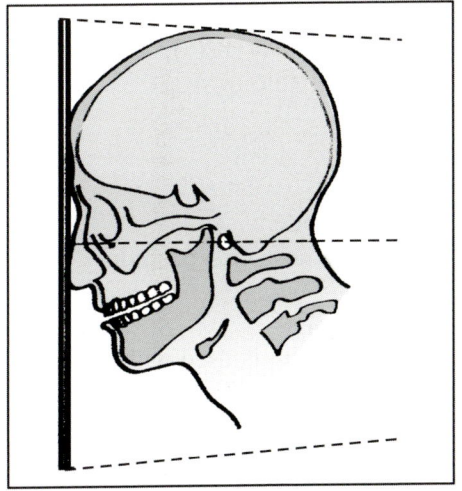 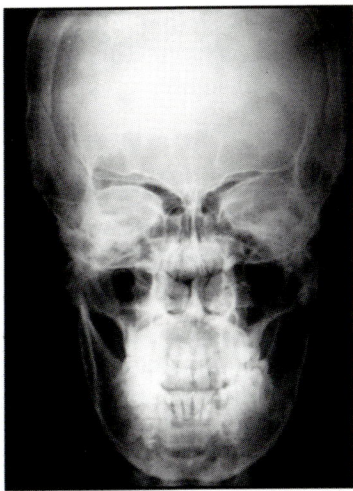

Fig. 3.57: Patient positioning for PA Caldwell view.

Fig. 3.58: PA Caldwell view.

The PA mandible view is similar to the Caldwell view except that the centering point is located at a level midway between the two rami. This enables better visualization of the mandible.

PA WATER'S VIEW

Indications

1. To study the maxillary sinuses.
2. To study the fractures involving the middle third of the facial skeleton.
3. To study the fractures involving the zygomatic arches and the orbits.
4. To study the deviated nasal septum.
5. To study the frontal and ethmoidal sinuses.
6. To study the coronoid process that is seen between the lateral wall of maxillary sinus and the zygomatic arch.

The drawback of Water's view is that it does not show the posterior wall of the maxillary sinus. To study this part, a submento vertex or a true lateral view is required. Also PA Water's view does not show the floor of the antrum clearly which can be visualized better on deep IOPA or topographic occlusal views (which are preferred to study oro-antral fistula).

If Water's view is made with the patient's mouth kept open, the sphenoid sinus can be seen. This is called the paranasal sinus (PNS) view as all the para nasal sinuses are visualized in this radiograph.

Head Position

   (i) MSP is perpendicular to the cassette.
  (ii) CML is at an angle of 45° to the cassette.
 (iii) The patient may be positioned in the nose-chin position.

Film and Cassette

An 8 × 10 inch or 10 × 12 inch high speed film is used with a suitable intensifying screen in a cassette.

Centering Point

The central ray passes through a point 2 inches above the external occipital protuberance (Fig. 3.59).

Angulation – The central ray is directed at 90° to the cassette. The resultant radiograph is shown in Fig. 3.60.

TFD – 3 feet
kVp – 80
mAS – 150

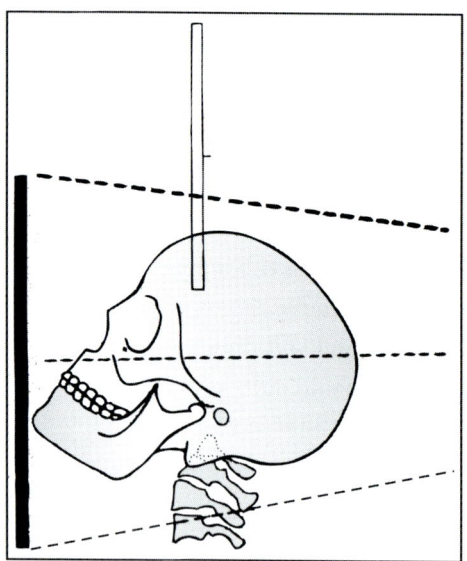

Fig. 3.59: Patient positioning for PA Water's view.

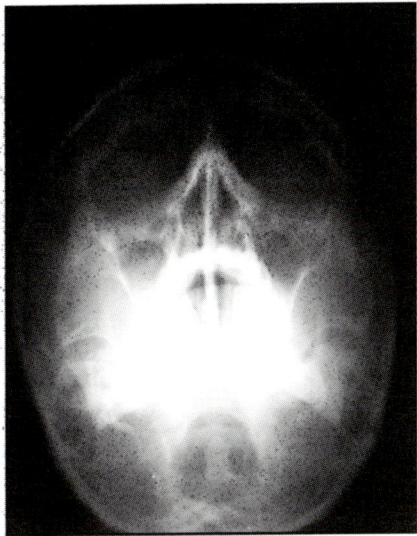

Fig. 3.60: PA Water's view.

PA ROTATED/TANGENTIAL VIEW

Indications

1. To study the calculus in parotid duct.
2. To study the displacement of condyle.

The patient's head is rotated in order to make the long axis of the condyle parallel to the cassette. In doing so the ramus becomes perpendicular to the cassette and the central ray passes tangential to the ramus. In such a position, the ramus and the condyle resemble the letter 'T'.

Head Position

The head is rotated to the side of interest by 20°.

Film and Cassette

An 8 × 10 inch or 10 × 12 inch high speed film is used with a suitable intensifying screen in a cassette.

Centering Point

The central ray passes through the angle of the mandible of the side of interest.

Angulation – The central ray is directed at 90° to the cassette.

TFD – 3 feet

kVp – 80

mAS – 150

REVERSE TOWNE'S VIEW

Indications

    1. To study condylar fracture and displacement.

    2. To study the continuity of zygomatic arch.

Head Position

    (i) MSP is perpendicular to the cassette.

    (ii) CML is at an angle of 90° to the cassette.

    (iii) The patient is positioned with his mouth open.

Film and Cassette

An 8 × 10 inch or 10 × 12 inch high speed film is used with suitable intensifying screens in a cassette.

Centering Point

The central ray passes through the nape of the neck and is directed 30° upward through the condyles. The resultant radiograph is shown in Fig. 3.61.

    TFD – 3 feet

    kVp – 80

    mAS – 150

SUBMENTO-VERTEX VIEW

Indications

    1. To study the fractures of zygomatic arch.

    2. To study the posterior wall of the maxillary sinus.

    3. To study fractures involving the base of the skull.

    4. To study sphenoidal air sinuses.

    5. To study the inclination of the condyles.

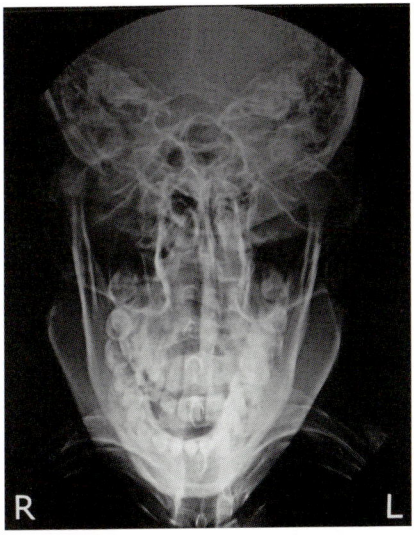

Fig. 3.61: Reverse Towne's view.

The jug handle view is a modified submento-vertex view that is made on a dental X-ray machine with a reduced exposure to give a clear picture of the zygomatic arches.

Head Position (Fig. 3.62)

(i) MSP is perpendicular to the cassette.

(ii) CML is parallel to the cassette. This is achieved by hyperextending the patient's neck. Care must be taken in doing so in a patient with

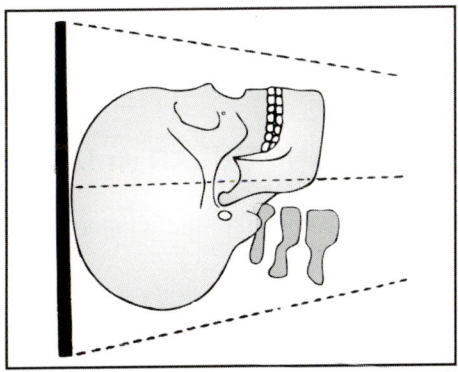

Fig. 3.62: Patient positioning for submento-vertex view.

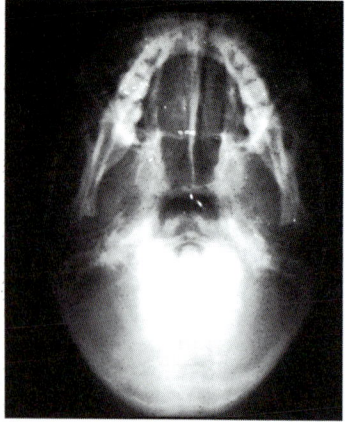

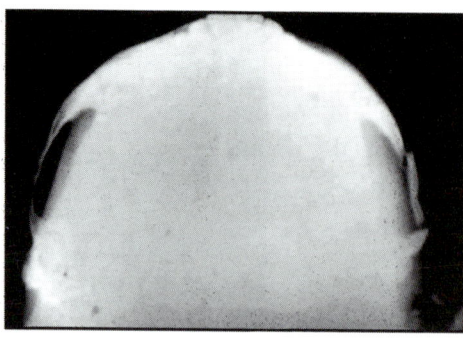

Fig. 3.64: A jug handle view showing fracture of the zygomatic arch.

Fig. 3.63: A submento-vertex view.

trauma to the neck and this view is contraindicated in a patient with suspected fractures of the odontoid peg.

Film and Cassette

An 8 × 10 inch high speed film is used with suitable intensifying screen in a cassette.

Centering Point

The central ray passes through a point 1.5 inches below the symphysis menti through the MSP.

Angulation – The central ray is directed at 90° to the cassette.

TFD – 3 feet

kVp – 80

mAS – 150

TEMPOROMANDIBULAR RADIOGRAPHY

The various views that demonstrate the temporomandibular joint are as follows:

1. Trans-Cranial view/ Lindblom's view
2. Trans-Pharyngeal view/Mc Queen's view/Parma projection
3. Trans-Orbital view/Zimmer's view

4. Rotated lateral view
5. Submento-vertex view
6. PA Caldwell's view
7. OPG
8. Bregma-menton view
9. Serial arthrometry
10. Superior oblique technique
11. Collar radiography
12. Tomography
13. Rotography
14. Arthrography
15. Stereoscopy
16. Arthroscopy
17. CT scans
18. MRI

TRANS-CRANIAL VIEW

Indications

1. To study the position of the condyles in the glenoid fossa.
2. To study the joint space, i.e. the space between the articulating surfaces of the glenoid fossa and the condyles for either partial or complete obliteration (ankylosis).

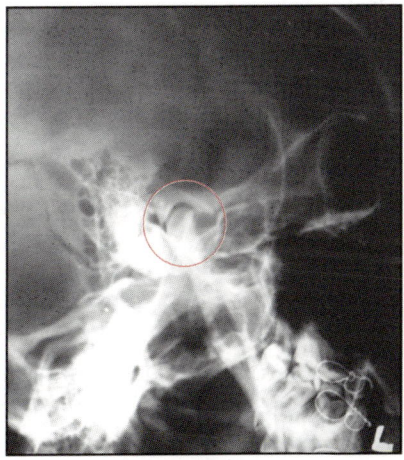

Fig. 3.65: A trans-cranial view (closed mouth).

3. To study antero-posterior mobility. (Hypermobility, i.e. dislocation and subluxation.)
4. To study osseous change such as flattening in arthritis.

The limitations of Trans-cranial view are:

(i) Subcondylar fractures are not seen on the Trans-cranial view because of superimposition of ipsilateral petrous bone and posterior clinoid process of sella turcica on the neck of the condyle.
(ii) The radiograph shows only the lateral part of the joint space.

Head Position

(i) MSP is parallel to the cassette.
(ii) The infraorbital line is perpendicular to the cassette.
(iii) The CML is parallel to the floor and the ear is held flat against the cassette.
(iv) This view is made both in open and in closed mouth positions.

Film and Cassette

A 5 × 7 inch or 8 × 10 inch high speed film with suitable double intensifying screens is used in a cassette.

Centering Point

Two inches above the external auditory meatus of the opposite side. The central ray is directed 25° downwards and 20° forwards towards the TMJ under study (Lindblom view)

TFD—6–8"
mA—10
kVp—65
Exposure time-1 second

TRANSPHARYNGEAL VIEW (Mc Queen's view)

Indications

1. To study the head and the neck of the condyle.
2. To study flattening of the condyle in rheumatoid arthritis and osteophytes in osteoarthritis. Osteophytes are small spike projections of bone.
3. To study elongated styloid process (Eagle's syndrome).

4. To study developmental anomalies affecting the condyle such as a bifid condyle.

5. To study fractures involving the neck of the condyle.

6. To study parotid gland sialography.

Head Position

(i) MSP is rotated 10 degrees to the side to be radiographed.

(ii) CML is parallel to the floor.

(iii) Patient is instructed to keep his mouth open. This increases the size of the window formed by the opposite side sigmoid notch and the zygomatic arch through which the central ray passes and also the condyle gets disengaged from the base of the skull, thereby preventing superimposition.

Cassette and the Film

A 5 × 7 inch or 8 × 10 inch high speed film with suitable double intensifying screen is used in a cassette.

TFD: 6 – 8 inches.

Centering Point

The CR passes through the sigmoid notch of the opposite side through the window formed by the condyle, coronoid process and the zygomatic arch of the opposite side. The point of intersection of a perpendicular drawn from the mid point of the CML to the ala tragus line marks the point of entry for the CR.

Angulation

The CR is directed 10° upward and 10° backwards towards the joint under study.

mA is 10

Exposure time: 0.5 second.

kVp: 65

In transpharyngeal view, the rays pass through the sigmoid notch of the opposite side, the pharynx and the condyle under study. The rays always pass below the base of the skull and hence this view is also called as *infra cranial view* or *lateral sigmoid view*.

Parma modification: It is a modification of the transpharyngeal view in which the cone is removed from the X-ray machine. This brings the

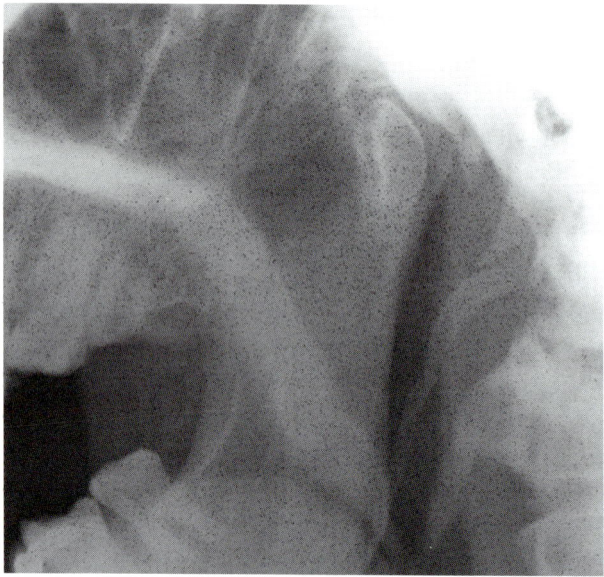

Fig. 3.66: A transpharyngeal view.

opposite side condyle closer to the tube giving rise to magnification and blurring which is desirable to view the condyle under study more clearly.

TRANSORBITAL VIEW

It is an A-P view of the TMJ which is also called as **Zimmerís view**

Indications

1. To study mediolateral displacement of the condyle.
2. To study superior surfaces of the condyle for osteophytes, etc.
3. To study the relationship of condyle to the articular eminence in the medio-lateral plane.

Head Position

(i) Patient's head is rotated 15° to the side to be radiographed.

(ii) CML is perpendicular to the cassette and parallel to the floor.

(iii) Patient is asked to open his mouth fully. (A wooden block may be used to keep the mouth open.) When the mouth is kept open, the condyles disengage from the glenoid fossa and super imposition of the articular eminence and mastoid process can be avoided.

Cassette and Film

A 5 × 7 inch or 8 × 10 inch high speed film with suitable double intensifying screens is used in a cassette.

Centering Point

The CR passes through the ipsilateral medial canthus of the eye anteriorly and directed towards the condyle under study.

Angulation

CR is directed with a 10° downward angulation and perpendicular to the cassette.

    TFD 15–20"

    mA is 10

    Exposure time: 1.5 seconds

    kVp: 65

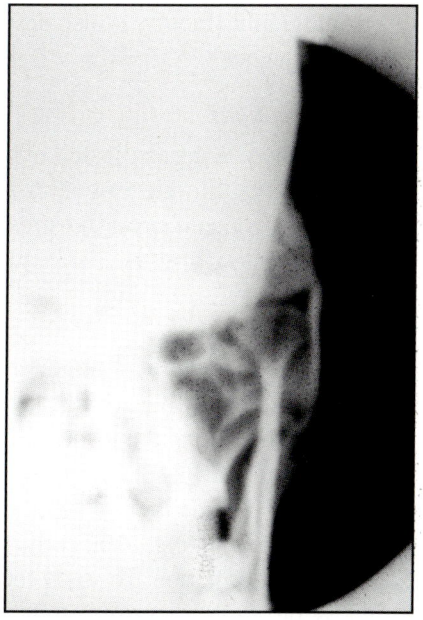

Fig. 3.67: A transorbital view.

SERIAL ARTHROMETRY

It is a transcranial view taken 3 times for each patient at open position, rest position, and closed position with an attempt to study accurate relationship between the condyle and the glenoid fossa. It is useful for treatment planning in patients with TMJ dysfunction and arthritis (with reduced or increased joint space).

ARTHROGRAPHY

A radiopaque contrast medium is injected in the superior compartment of the joint and trans-cranial view is made. Presence of a perforation in the meniscus can be identified if dye flows into the inferior compartment.

If series of radiographs are made the internal derangement of TMJ can be studied by viewing the position of the disc. This procedure is best carried out in operation theatres with fluoroscopic facility which permits the radiologist to ascertain correct placement of the needle in the joint space and also to prevent infections and other complications.

Tomographic facility is also desirable to appreciate the entire joint in a sectional manner.

Contraindications

Arthrography is contraindicated in acute inflammatory conditions of TMJ and in patients allergic to contrast media. A potential disadvantage of arthrography is that if excessive pressure is applied while injecting the dye, it can result into iatrogenic perforation of the disc.

TOMOGRAPHY

Tomography or body section radiography is the study of a layer within the body by intentionally blurring the layers above and below it. This is achieved by moving the film and the source synchronously in opposite direction so that one particular layer within the object called the focal plane remains sharp (Fig. 3.68). It is used to study the pathologies of TMJ, maxillary sinus, implant imaging when conventional radiography fails to reveal any significant information. To study the TMJ, a corrected tomography can be made by determining the angulation of the condyle using measurements made on a submento-vertex view. The patient is then positioned with the long axis of the condyle perpendicular to the film. (Rather than arbitrarily positioning with a 20° head rotation towards the side of interest.)

PANORAMIC RADIOGRAPHY

Orthopantomograph (OPG) is a curvilinear variant of conventional tomography which is based on the principle of reciprocal movement of the film and the source around the central plane called the image layer. This is called the focal trough which is a 3D curved zone located within the object whose image is seen clearly on the radiograph.

The X-ray source rotates around three centers of rotation during the scanning.

Indications

1. To evaluate cases of trauma for fractures and dislocations.
2. To study and locate impacted, unerupted and supernumerary teeth.
3. To study the alignment of teeth for orthodontic treatment planning.
4. To study developmental anomalies affecting the teeth and jaws.
5. To study cysts and tumors occurring in the jaws.

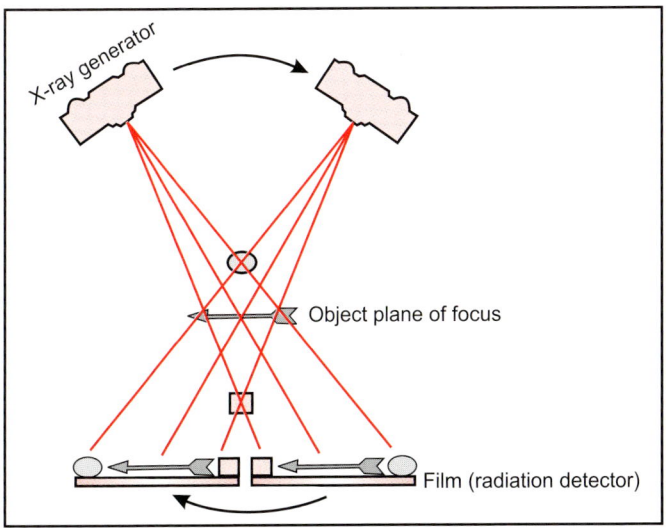

Straight arrow is the plane of focus so it remains clear.
Circle and square are out of the plane so they are blurred because they are imaged across the radiation detector.

Fig. 3.68: Principle of tomography.

6. To study the TMJ and maxillary sinuses.

7. To study parotid sialogram.

The advantages of OPG

(i) The entire jaws (maxilla and mandible) can be studied in one film.

(ii) It is a relatively simple procedure.

(iii) Minimum patient cooperation is required as opposed to IOPA views where problems such as trismus and gagging are encountered.

(iv) The entire procedure requires less than 5 minutes as compared to a full mouth radiographic examination which requires about 15 minutes.

(v) Radiation dose is less as compared to full mouth radiography because:

(a) OPG utilizes slit beam collimation (2 mm × 30 mm).

(b) X-rays are directed 7° upwards and the body is relatively unexposed.

(vi) An OPG is better for patient education purpose at it can be easily explained by the doctor and understood by the patient.

The disadvantages of OPG

The image quality is inferior as compared to IOPA views because of:

 (a) Magnification

 (b) Geometric distortion

 (c) Unsharpness

These defects are due to the tomographic process (movement) and also because of:

 (a) External placement of film.

 (b) Increased object film distance.

 (c) Increased speed of the film and intensifying screen (due to large grain size).

Head Position

 (i) MSP is perpendicular to the floor. If it is tilted to one side, it will cause uneven magnification of the image.

 (ii) FHP is parallel to the floor. In other words, the occlusal plane is at an angle of 20–30° with the floor.

 (iii) If the chin is excessively tipped upwards, it will cause flattening/inversion of the occlusal plane on the radiograph. Also the shadow of the hard palate superimposes over the root apices of the maxillary teeth and the condyles may be lost laterally.

 (iv) If the chin is tipped excessively downwards, the occlusal plane appears curved on the image. Also superimposition of the upper and lower teeth may take place and the condyles may be lost superiorly.

 (v) The patient's neck should be kept straight and should not slump because then the shadow of the spine will superimpose on the symphyseal region, thereby obscuring important details in this region.

 (vi) If the patient is positioned too anteriorly in the focal trough, it will result in narrowing of the anterior teeth on the radiograph. While if placed too posteriorly, there will be unwanted widening of the images of the teeth.

 (vii) The midline should be aligned properly with the bite block. If not, there will be widening of the teeth and ramus on the side which is away from the film and narrowing of teeth and ramus on the side towards the film.

(viii) The patient is instructed to hold the tongue against the palate to avoid the superimposition of the air space between the tongue and the palate on the periapical region of the maxillary teeth.

Cassette and the Film

A 6 × 12 inch high speed film with suitable double intensifying screen is used in a cassette. Some of the cassettes used in certain machines are curved/flexible.

Angulation

The angulations of the CR are pre-adjusted in the machine. The central ray is directed about 5–7° upwards. The machine moves about three centers of rotations, one each to scan the right and left side of the posterior region of the jaws up to the premolars and one for the anterior region.

kVp: 68

mA: 10

Exposure time: 18 seconds.

Notes

CHAPTER 4

Digital Imaging

With the rapid development in the field of computers and technology, newer methods of image acquisition and processing are available. These systems utilize electronic media to record the images and advanced computer software to process the acquired image and also modify it according to our needs.

Advantages of digital imaging systems

1. Chemical processing of the films is not required. As a result of this the detrimental effect of improper processing on the image quality can be avoided.

2. Waste products resulting from chemical processing and lead foils present in the film packet which may pose an environmental hazard are safely avoided.

3. The acquired images can be modified to obtain the desirable density and contrast.

4. The exposure latitude is higher in digital imaging as compared to the conventional films.

5. Images can be archived without the loss of their quality and retrieved as and when required.

6. Images can be transmitted via electronic media.

Disadvantages of digital imaging system

1. The expenditure involved in setting up a digital imaging system is quite high.

2. The image receptors are vulnerable to the effects of rough handling. Once damaged, they are expensive to replace.

3. The image receptors are bulky, rigid and cumbersome. The patient finds it difficult to tolerate the rigid sensor in mouth as compared to the conventional film.

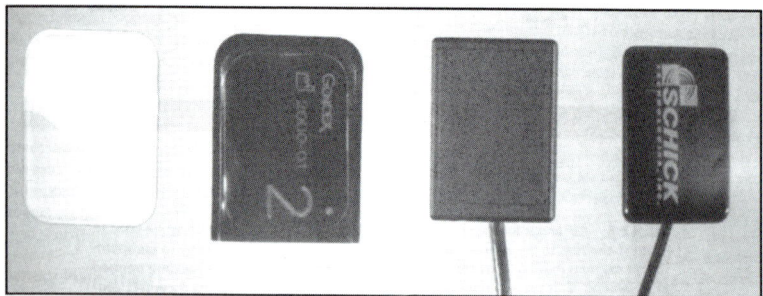

Fig. 4.1: Different image receptors –IOPA film, PSP plate and CCD.

4. The resolution of images acquired with a digital system is inferior to conventional films based images.
5. At a time not more than two to three teeth can be studied with digital image receptors.
6. Since the images can be manipulated, the authenticity of the images and their validity as evidence in a medio-legal case are questionable.

The digital images are different from the conventional images in the following manner. In a conventional film based image, the difference in the density at different places on the film due to the size and distribution of the silver halide particles forms the image. In a digital system, the image is divided into many small picture elements called pixels. Each pixel is assigned a numerical value based upon shade of gray corresponding to the respective pixel. The numbers range from 0 to 255, where, 0 represents completely black areas and 255 represents completely white areas on the radiograph. Each pixel has a row and column co-ordinate that helps to identify its unique location in the matrix.

DIGITAL IMAGE DETECTORS

The three main types of digital image recording devices are:
    A. Charged-coupled device (CCD).
    B. Complimentary metal oxide semiconductors (CMOS).
    C. Photostimulable phosphor plates (PSP).

Other image recording devices include the Bulk charge modulating device (BCMD), Thin film transistor (TFT), Flat plane detectors.

A. Charged-coupled Device (CCD)

(i) The CCD is formed of n-p silicon sandwich to which electrodes are attached (Fig. 4.2).

(ii) The surface of the silicon is coated with a scintillating material such as gadolinium oxysulphide or cesium oxide, since the device is more sensitive to light.

(iii) When radiation falls on the detector, the covalent bond between the silicon atoms are broken and electron-hole pairs are produced. The number of hole pairs produced is proportional to the amount of radiation incident on the device (Fig. 4.3).

(iv) The electrons are attracted towards the most positive potential within the device where they create "***charge packets***" corresponding to each pixel. Each charge packet represents the latent image.

(v) When the image is read out, the charges are transferred from one pixel to the other in a ***bucket brigade*** like fashion.

(vi) When the charges reach the end of the row, it is transferred to a read out amplifier and transmitted as a voltage to the *analog to digital converter (ADC)*. The voltage from each pixel is sampled and assigned a numerical value which represents its grey scale.

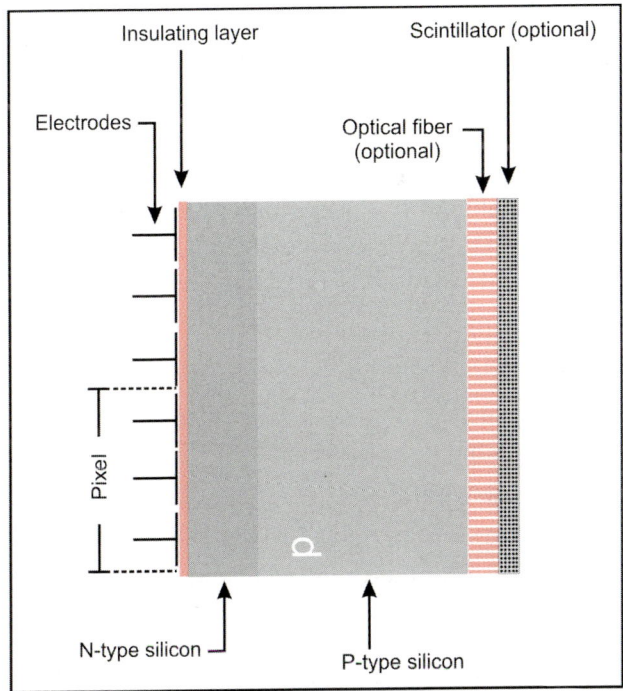

Fig. 4.2: Diagram showing the construction of CCD.

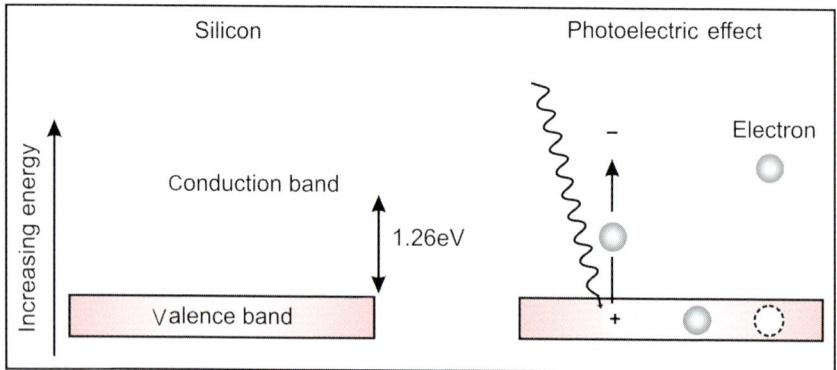

Fig. 4.3: Formation of electron-hole pair in a CCD.

B. Complimentary Metal Oxide Semiconductors (CMOS)

The CMOS system also uses a silicon semiconductor like the CCD. The basic mechanism of formation of a latent image is same as with a CCD. However, the manner in which the charges are read is different from that in a CCD. In a CMOS, each pixel is connected directly to a transistor and charges are read directly. The data undergoes *analog to digital conversion (ADC)* and specific numbers are assigned to the pixels depending upon their density.

C. Photostimulable Phosphor Plates (PSP)

The PSP systems are different from CCD/CMOS in construction and working. The material used is a photostimulable phosphor plate made up of "Europium doped" Barium flurohalide. Barium combines with the halides to form a crystal, while addition of Europium creates imperfections in the lattice.

Principle and Working

1. The PSP plate absorbs the radiant energy from the X-rays and releases it in the form of visible light when stimulated (Fig. 4.4).
2. When exposed to radiation, europium (Eu^{+2}) releases e^-.
   $$Eu^{+2} + X\text{-rays} \longrightarrow Eu^{+3} + e^-$$
3. The electrons which are released migrate to the halogen valencies called F centers in the flurohalide crystals and get trapped in a metastable form. The amount of electrons entrapped is proportional to the amount of radiation incident on the PSP plate and the F centers represent the latent image site.

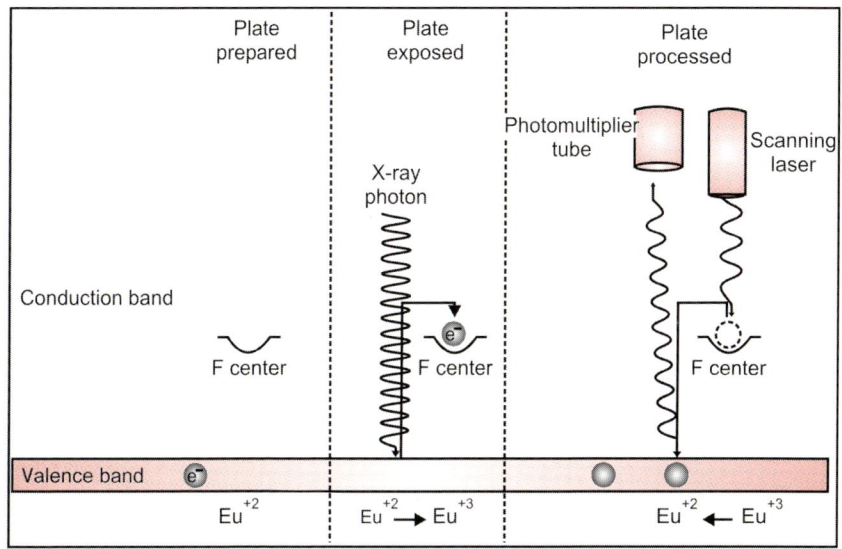

Fig. 4.4: Working of PSP plates.

4. When the exposed plate having the latent image site is stimulated by light of wavelength 600 nm, the F centers release the electrons to the conduction band thereby liberating energy in the form of visible green light.

5. This green light after passing through red filter to remove the stimulant red light enters a photomultiplier tube that converts light into voltage signal.

6. The voltage then undergoes *analog to digital conversion (ADC)* to form an image.

DIGITAL SUBTRACTION RADIOGRAPHY

Digital subtraction radiography is a technique which allows the amount of background information to be reduced and thus permit the observer to concentrate on the tissue changes that have taken place by subtracting the normal anatomic structures that have not changed between the radiographic examinations. Two important prerequisites to be performed for digital subtraction radiography are:

(i) Both the images must be obtained with the same projection geometry. To obtain images with the same projection geometry, standardization of patient positioning with the use of stabilizing devices and film holding devices can be used. A stored video image of the patient may be taken during the first radiographic examination and used as a guide to position the patient during the subsequent sessions.

(ii) Both the images must have the same density and contrast. With the availability of digital systems, the contrast and density of the two radiographs can be matched and digital subtraction can be easily performed.

The computer subtracts the digital gray scale value for each pixel to obtain a subtracted image. In doing so all the normal structures are subtracted and the change that has occurred in the tissues becomes apparent. Digital subtraction radiography is useful in post treatment evaluation of patients who have undergone periodontal surgery and in sialography.

SUGGESTED READING AND REFERENCES

1. Oral Radiology. Principles and Interpretation: White & Pharoah - 5th edition.

2. Essentials of Dental Radiography and Radiology. Eric Whaites, 3rd edition.

3. Application of Digital Imaging Modality for Dentistry. DCNA April 2000.

CHAPTER 5

Principles of Radiographic Interpretation

PRINCIPLES OF RADIOGRAPHIC INTERPRETATION

The term to interpret means to explain. The term radiographic interpretation means explanation of the various features of the radiographic image. Radiographic interpretation involves a step by step analysis of the acquired image to arrive at a conclusion. In order to enable the radiologist to interpret the radiograph correctly, the following are some of the important requirements.

1. The correct choice and number of radiographic views must be available to study the suspected pathology. In doing so the radiologist must take into account the advantages and limitations of each radiographic technique, e.g. attempting to diagnose early proximal caries on OPG may yield an erroneous result.

2. The radiographs must be of good quality. Distorted, excessively dark/light radiographs may not be suitable for interpretation.

3. Ideal viewing conditions must be present while examining the radiographs. The ideal conditions include:

    (a) Reduced ambient light in the room.

    (b) IOPA radiographs should be mounted in a film holder.

    (c) The light from the view box must be of uniform intensity throughout the viewing surface.

    (d) The size of the view box must accommodate the size of the film.

    (e) An intense light source may be required for viewing dark radiographs.

    (f) A magnifying lens must be used to see the minute details.

Before setting out to do radiographic interpretation one must be fully aware of the inherent limitations of radiography (such as 2-D image of a

3-D object), must have adequate knowledge of anatomy and pathology, and how the pathology alters the anatomical structures, and how in turn this process modifies the radiographic appearance.

IMAGE ANALYSIS

Intraoral Images

While interpreting IOPA views, the radiographic findings in each tooth may be studied and reported under the following headings:

 (i) Crown: Study the developmental defects, caries, attrition, abrasion, fractures, etc.

 (ii) Roots: Study the number, shape and size of the roots. Examine carefully for the presence of dilacerations, root resorption, ankylosis, incompletely formed apices, etc.

 (iii) Pulp chamber: Examine the size of the pulp chamber, involvement of one or more walls by caries, presence of pulp stones, etc.

 (iv) Root canals: Study the number of canals in the roots, their shape and size, which may be valuable in planning endodontic treatment.

 (v) Lamina dura: Discontinuity in the lamina dura may be sign of periapical disease. When generalized loss of lamina dura is seen, appropriate differential diagnosis must be considered.

 (vi) Periodontal ligament space: Observe the space for presence of widening, disappearance, etc. which indicate a disease process.

 (vii) Alveolar crest: Observe the level and form of the crest. A normal alveolar crest is sharp in the anterior region and blunt with sharp edges in the posterior region. Deviation from the normal finding may indicate periodontal disease.

 (viii) Periapical region: Observe the peri apex of each tooth to detect abscess, granuloma, cysts, PCD, etc.

The anatomical landmarks and artifacts that have appeared on the radiographs must be noted carefully and should not be mistaken for pathological findings.

Extraoral Radiographs

While interpreting extraoral radiographs for intraosseous pathologies, the following 5 steps may be followed.

STEP 1 – Localizing the abnormality.

(a) The anatomic location and extent of the lesion must be determined. If the lesion may be localized, it may be unilateral or bilateral. Sometimes anatomical variations may be localized and mimic a pathology. In such cases the variation is usually bilaterally symmetrical. If the lesion appears to be generalized and involving both the jaws, then in such cases a systemic pathology affecting the bone should be considered, e.g. metabolic or endocrine disorders, Paget's disease, metastatic disease.

(b) The position of the lesion in the jaws must be ascertained. The point of origin or the epicenter should be identified which gives important clue regarding the nature of the lesion. If the epicenter is located above the mandibular canal, the lesion is usually odontogenic in origin, e.g. radicular cyst, if it originates within the canal, it is usually of neurovascular nature. Lesions having an epicenter below the canal are likely to be of non odontogenic in origin, e.g. Stafne's bone cyst.

Certain lesions tend to favour certain specific locations, e.g. the epicenter of giant cell granuloma is usually anterior to the first molars in the mandible and anterior to the canines in the maxilla. Osteomyelitis frequently affects the mandible. Periapical cemental dysplasias are generally seen in the mandibular anterior region.

(c) Single or multifocal lesions: Certain lesions like PCD, OKC, metastatic malignancies, leukemic infiltrates have a tendency to occur as multifocal lesions.

STEP 2 – Assessing the periphery of the lesion.

Margins of the lesions affecting the jaws may be well-defined or ill-defined. When an imaginary line can be drawn confidently to limit the lesion, it may be called as a well-defined margin.

Well-defined margin may be further categorized as:

(a) Punched out margin which has a sharp margin, but no bone reaction is apparent immediately adjacent to the lesion, e.g. multiple myeloma.

(b) Corticated margin which has a thin radiopaque line of reactive bone at the periphery, e.g. cysts.

(c) Sclerotic margin which is a thick radiopaque border of reactive bone not uniform in width, e.g. PCD.

(d) A radiopaque lesion may have a radiolucent halo around it which represents the soft tissue capsule, e.g. odontomes.

Ill-defined margins appear as:

(a) Blending margins due to gradual transition between the normal and abnormal bony trabeculae. The focus of attention in a blending margin is on the trabeculae.

(b) Invasive/permeative margins are seen with malignant tumors where the lesion grows around the existing trabeculae producing finger like extensions into the periphery.

STEP 3 – Analyzing the internal structure of the lesion.

Based upon the appearance of the internal structure, the lesions may be categorized as radiolucent, radiopaque and mixed lesions.

(a) Residual bone inside the lesion may resemble septa and give rise to a multilocular appearance, e.g. ameloblastoma, OKC, aneurysmal bone cyst.

(b) Abnormal bony trabeculae may be arranged as numerous, fine, short patterns giving rise to a ground glass appearance in fibrous dysplasia.

(c) Presence of tooth or tooth like substance may be identified inside the lesion as in dentigerous cyst, ameloblastomas, OKC, etc.

STEP 4 – Analyzing the effect of the lesion on the adjacent structures.

Space occupying lesions are those which grow by slowly creating space for themselves by displacing the adjacent teeth or landmarks.

(a) Lesions having epicenter above the crown of the teeth may push the tooth apically.

(b) Lesions which grow inside the papilla push the tooth coronally, e.g. leukemia, Langerhan's cell histiocytosis, lymphoma.

(c) Cysts and benign tumors cause displacement of the canal inferiorly.

(d) Fibrous dysplasia causes displacement of canal superiorly.

(e) Root resorption is usually caused by cyst and benign tumors, and occasionally by malignant tumor. The resorption caused by a slowly growing benign process appears as a smooth cuplike resorption, while malignant tumors cause irregular spiked resorption.

STEP 5 – Formulating the radiographic diagnosis.

After analyzing the lesion thoroughly, a radiographic diagnosis may be formulated. The first step this is to find out if the radiographic finding is actually a lesion or is just a variation of normal. If a lesion is identified, it must be identified as a developmental or acquired lesion. An acquired lesion must be further categorized based upon its nature as a lesion that may be an inflammatory, neoplastic, traumatic, etc.

The radiographic sieve as shown in Fig 5.1 can serve as a guide to arrive at the right radiographic diagnosis.

As quoted by H.M.Worth, three main changes can be seen in the radiographic appearance of any bony condition. They are:

1. Demineralization/decalcification/rarefaction of the bone causing thinning of the trabeculae.

2. Destruction of the trabeculae, so that the bone appears completely radiolucent.

3. Condensation/sclerosis: More and more bone may get deposited into the marrow spaces by a mechanism called appositional bone deposition causing a radiopacity within the bone.

The radiographic report: A detailed radiographic report which must have the following details must be given to the patient.

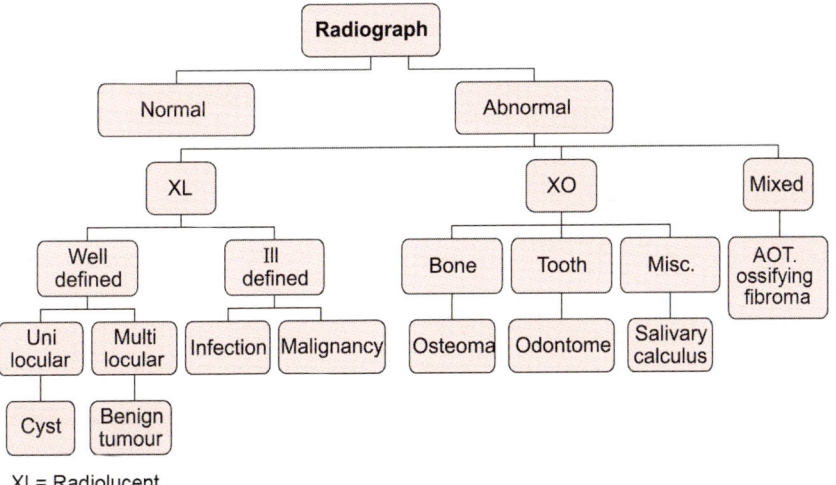

XL= Radiolucent
XO=Radiopaque

Fig. 5.1: The radiographic sieve; XL = Radiolucent, XO = Radiopaque.

1. Patient's name and general information.
2. Name of the referring clinician.
3. A brief clinical history of the patient.
4. Details of the imaging procedure that was performed.

5. Radiographic findings.
6. Radiographic impression.

The report should conclude with the radiologist's comment on further evaluation and must be duly signed by him.

SUGGESTED READING AND REFERENCES

1. Oral Radiology—Principles and Interpretation: White and Pharoah, 5th edition.
2. Essentials of Dental Radiography and Radiology—Eric Whaites, 3rd edition.
3. Principles and Practice of Radiographic Interpretation—H.M. Worth.
4. The Clinical Approach to Radiographic Diagnosis—DCNA Jan 1994.

Notes

CHAPTER 6

Dental Caries and Periapical Lesions

DENTAL CARIES

Definition

Dental caries is defined as a progressive microbial disease of the calcified tissues of the teeth characterized by demineralization of the inorganic portion of the teeth and degeneration of the organic matrix.

Classification of Dental Caries

Based on the surfaces affected, caries can be classified as:

  (i) Pit and fissure caries

  (ii) Smooth surface caries

Based on the tissues affected, caries can be classified as:

  (i) Enamel caries

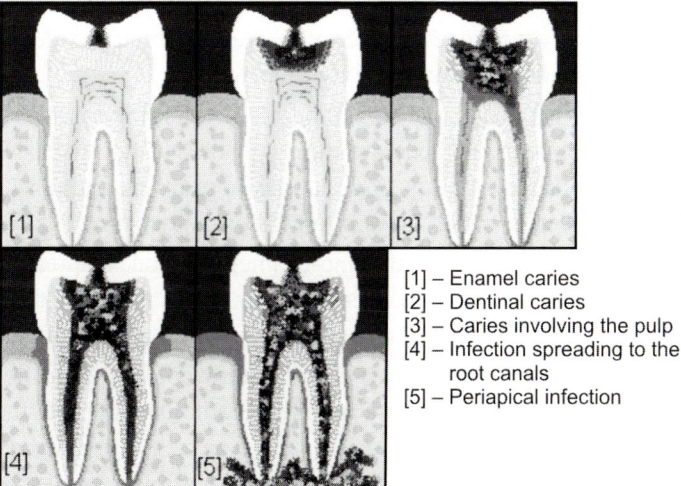

[1] – Enamel caries
[2] – Dentinal caries
[3] – Caries involving the pulp
[4] – Infection spreading to the root canals
[5] – Periapical infection

Fig. 6.1: Progression of dental caries.

(ii) Dentinal caries

(iii) Cemental/root surface caries

Limitations of Radiography in Diagnosing Dental Caries

(i) Radiographs provide a 2-D image of a 3-D structure. Hence buccal caries which may be away from the pulp chamber may appear to involve the pulp on the radiograph.

(ii) At least 30% calcium salts must have been removed from the tooth for the change to become apparent on the radiograph. In other words very early incipient lesions may be missed out on the radiographs.

(iii) The exact extent of caries cannot be visualized on the radiograph because a zone of demineralization at the advancing front of the lesion is not apparent. Hence, it is wise not to comment about the involvement of pulp by the caries using radiographic findings alone.

(iv) Occlusal caries cannot be detected in their early stages.

(v) Secondary caries occurring under the restorations may not be seen.

Radiographic Appearance of Caries

1. Radiographically caries appears as a dark shadow.

2. In the initial stages caries cannot be seen on the radiographs because sufficient decalcification has not taken place at that time.

3. The earliest change noticed in the area of decalcification is in the form of loss of homogenecity of enamel.

4. As caries spreads, the area of decalcification increases and darker areas appear on the radiographs where the tooth has actually disintegrated. At this stage, caries appears as irregular area of radiolucency which fades into the normal dentine (Fig. 6.2).

5. As caries reaches the dentino-enamel junction, it spreads rapidly over the surface of the underlying dentine undermining the enamel. On clinical examination such a tooth has a dark opaque hue.

6. Occlusal caries appears as a dark shadow under the enamel cap of the crown. It is seen as a triangular radiolucency with the broad base towards the DEJ.

7. Buccal or lingual caries appear as sharply defined radiolucent areas, round or elliptical in shape (Fig. 6.3). Buccal and lingual caries

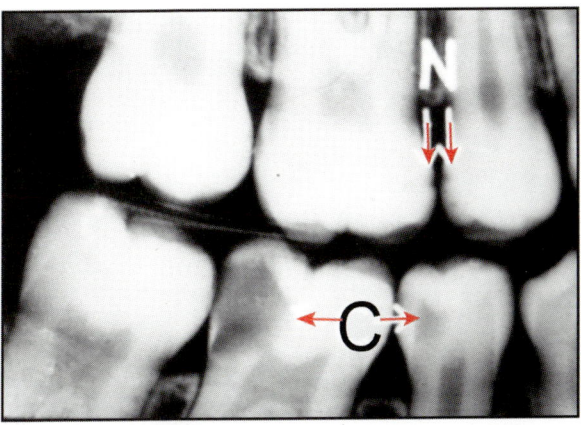

Fig. 6.2: Bitewing radiograph showing proximal caries [C] and early carries (N).

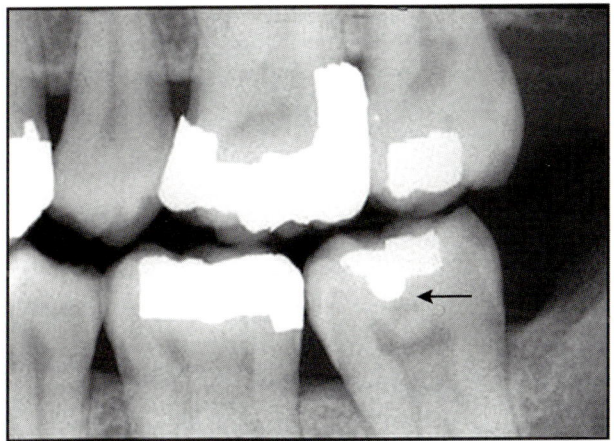

Fig. 6.3: Radiograph showing buccal/lingual caries (arrow).

cannot be differentiated from each other on a periapical radiograph. Also they may superimpose on the DEJ giving an erroneous appearance of occlusal caries. Occlusal caries however are more extensive and do not have well-defined margins.

8. Secondary caries appears as an arrow-shaped area of radiolucency under the restoration (Fig. 6.4).

Radiographic Classification of Proximal Caries

C1 – Caries penetrating less than half way into the enamel surface.

C2 – Caries penetrating more than half way into the enamel, but not affecting the dentine.

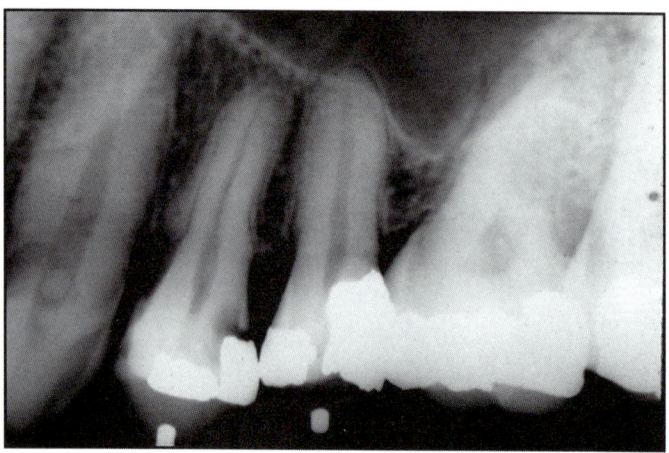

Fig. 6.4: Radiograph showing secondary caries in the first premolar.

C3 – Caries involving the dentino-enamel junction, but less than half way to the pulp.

C4 – Caries penetrating more than half way to the pulp.

Differential Diagnosis of Dental Caries (Shadows mistaken for caries)

1. **Erosion cavity:** It has sharp margins as compared to dental caries.
2. **Non-opaque fillings:** Well-defined margins of the prepared cavity are visible on the X-ray (Fig. 6.5).
3. **Internal resorption:** It appears as well demarcated, punched out radiolucency which is continuous with the root canal or pulp chamber (Fig. 6.6).
4. **External resorption:** It appears in areas that are covered with bone or soft tissue and it is well demarcated.
5. **Hypoplastic enamel:** It is a well demarcated radiolucency with nodules of enamel in between. The condition is usually bilaterally symmetrical (Fig. 6.7).
6. **Radiation caries:** Refer to radiation hazards (Fig. 6.8).
7. If the tooth is broad buccally, and narrow palatally, less radiopaque material will be available at the periphery, giving rise to a uniform, well demarcated radiolucency resembling caries.
8. **Cervical burn out:** Cervical burn out appears as a band-shaped radiolucency at the cemento-enamel junction (Fig. 6.9). The

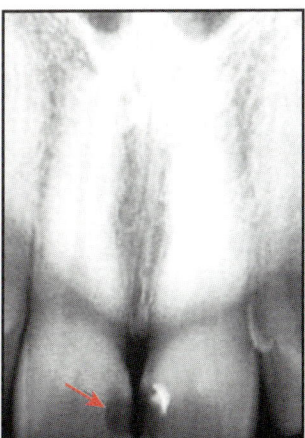

Fig. 6.5: Radiograph showing non-opaque fillings (arrow) with well-defined margins.

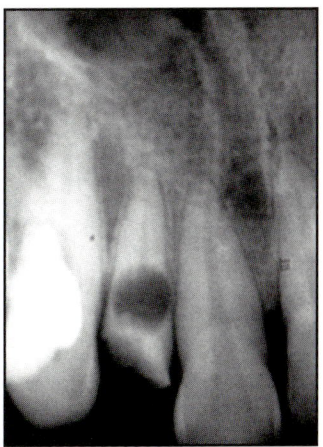

Fig. 6.6: Radiograph showing internal resorption in the lateral incisor.

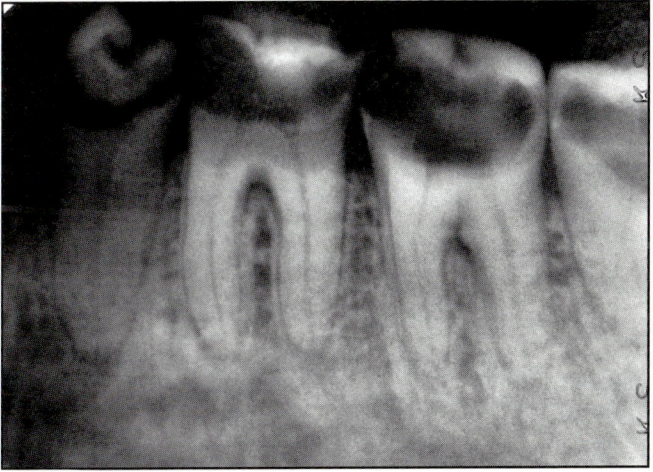

Fig. 6.7: Radiograph of hypoplastic teeth resembling caries.

coronal portion of the dentin is covered with enamel and the root portion is covered with cementum and alveolar bone. But at the cemento-enamel junction, the dentin has a very thin covering of enamel and cementum. In other words, at the cemento-enamel junction, the amount of radiopaque material available is less and hence when the radiograph is made, band or wedge-shaped radiolucency appears at the cemento-enamel junction which is termed as cervical burnout.

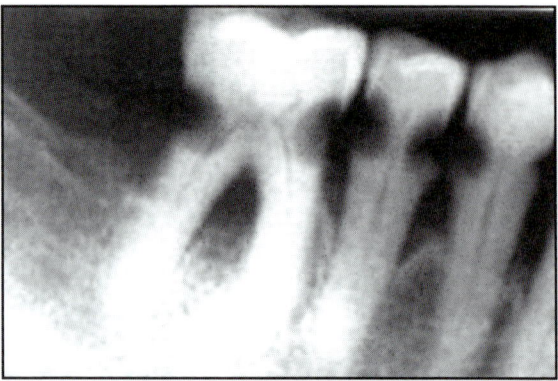

Fig. 6.8: Radiograph showing punched out appearance of radiation caries.

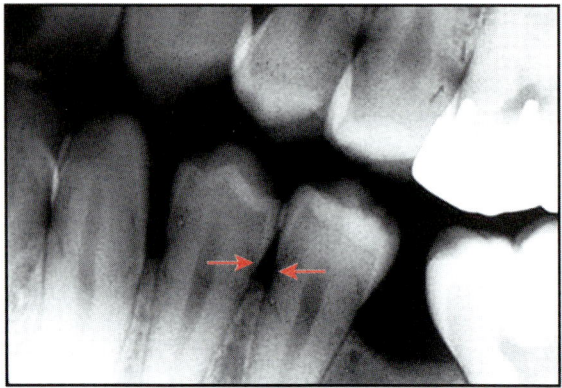

Fig. 6.9: Radiograph showing cervical burnout (arrows).

9. **Mach band effect:** At the junction of two structures which have sharply defined density difference, the area just adjacent to the high density structure appears as low density. This is an optical illusion and is known as *mach band*. Such an optical illusion may be seen on dental radiographs at the junction of enamel and dentine, where dentine appears as an area of low density adjacent to the enamel. This may be mistaken for caries.

PERIAPICAL LESIONS

Infection can reach the apex of the tooth either through the root canals or the periodontal ligament or through the medium of blood (*anachoresis*). The most common cause of periapical lesions is the sequelae of dental caries (Fig. 6.1). When caries is very deep and reaches the pulp, it sets up an intense inflammatory reaction associated with throbbing pain called pulpits. Excessive exudates and increase in vasculature gives rise to strangulation of the blood vessels at the apical foramen. This happens because the inflamed pulp is surrounded on all sides by the tooth wall and the exudate has no place to expand and exerts intense pressure on the neurovascular bundle at the apical foramen. This strangulation gives rise to decreased blood supply to the tooth and in due course of time the tooth becomes non vital. The infection now reaches the periapical area.

Cervical burnout	Caries
It is located closer to the alveolar crest.	It is located closer to the contact point.
It appears as a band-shaped radiolucency.	It appears as an irregular radiolucency.
It appears well demarcated on the radiograph.	It appears as a diffuse radiolucency on the radiograph.
Cervical burn out is seen well if horizontal angulation is incorrect.	Dental caries is seen well if horizontal angulation is correct.
The knife edge shape of the enamel at the CEJ remains intact.	The knife edge shape of the enamel at the CEJ is effaced.

Acute Apical Abscess

During the initial stages the inflammatory exudate is present in the bone marrow spaces and enough calcium is not removed from the trabeculae and therefore radiograph may not show any changes. The initial radiographic finding is a widening of the periodontal ligament space which may be due to:

(i) Escape of exudate into the periodontal ligament space causing slight elevation of the tooth in the socket.

(ii) Resorption of root.

(iii) Resorption of the apical bone.

Periapical Lesions appearing as Radiolucencies are:

(a) Abscess
(b) Granuloma
(c) Radicular cyst
(d) Periapical cemental dysplasia (first stage)
(e) Periapical lesion at the apex of a treated tooth
(f) Apical scar

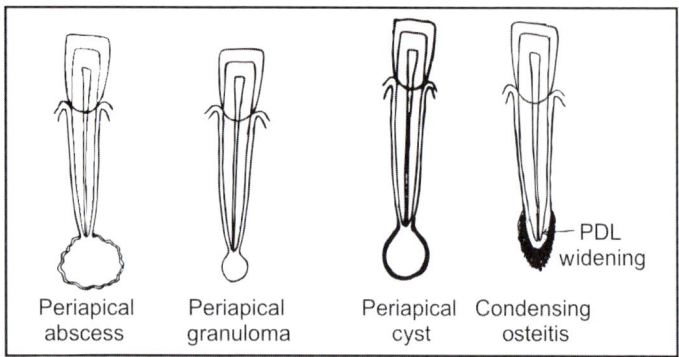

Fig. 6.10: Diagram showing the periapical changes in various lesions.

(g) Apisectomy wound

(h) Secondary infection

(i) Residual infection at the site of an extracted tooth

Periapical lesions appearing as radiopacities:

(a)   Condensing osteitis

(b)   Periapical cemental dysplasia (mature stage)

The periapical changes associated with an abscess, cyst, granuloma and condensing osteitis are represented in Fig. 6.10.

Periapical Abscess

When the virulence of the organism is more or if the host resistance is lowered, the organisms multiply rapidly and give rise to suppuration in the apical area. As this acute lesion becomes more chronic, it appears on the radiograph as a diffuse radiolucency with irregular margins which gradually merges with the surrounding bone (Fig. 6.11). The lamina dura of the offending tooth is discontinuous in the periapical area.

Periapical Granuloma

When the resistance of the host is good or if the virulence of the organisms is low, there is an effort on the part of the body to wall off the infection thereby giving rise to a granuloma. This is usually smaller in size than a cyst and unlike a cyst appears as a well circumscribed radiolucency without any corticated margin. The lamina dura of the associated tooth is missing around the apex (Fig. 6.12b).

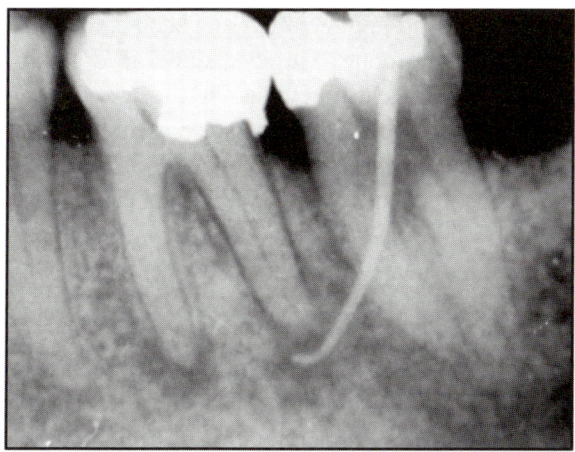

Fig. 6.11: Radiograph showing periapical abscess in the first molar. A GP point passed through the sinus tract points to the apex of the offending tooth.

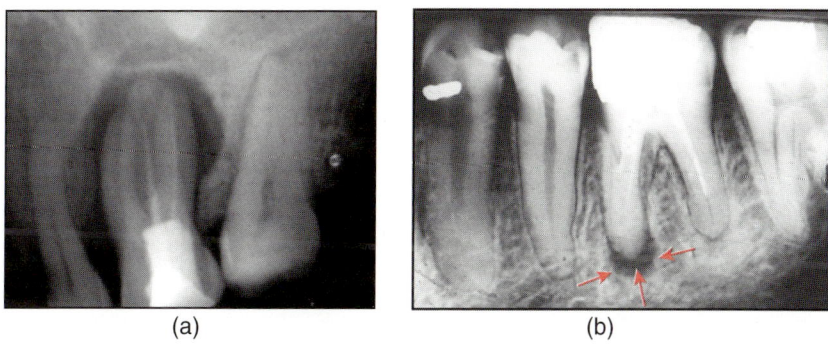

(a)   (b)

Fig 6.12: (a) Radiograph of an endodontically treated tooth showing periapical abscess indicating an endo-periocomplex disease, (b) Radiograph showing periapical granuloma (arrows).

Periapical Cyst

The periapical cyst develops in a granuloma from the epithelial cell rests of Malassez. The development of a cyst takes place in three stages: initiation, cyst formation and enlargement of the cyst. As the epithelial cells in the granuloma proliferate, the central cells degenerate to form a cystic cavity that expands by progressive accumulation of fluids.

The cyst appears on the radiograph (Figs 6.13 and 6.14) as a round or oval-shaped radiolucency surrounded by a thin white line called a corticated or hyperostotic border. This cortex is nothing but the condensation of bone due to the pressure exerted by the fluid filled lesion. The cyst may cause expansion of the cortex and might exhibit egg shell crackling as a result of excessive thinning of the bone. The cyst undergoes expansion by sub periosteal deposition of bone. Sometimes the cyst grows faster than bone formation giving rise to an area where sub periosteal bone is missing. It is at this site that egg shell crackling can be elicited. Sometimes the cyst may escape out on to the soft tissues and will show fluctuation. The radiograph then shows a window like appearance within the cystic lumen. After treating the cyst, the bony defect heals slowly and produces a sunray appearance on the radiograph (Fig. 6.15).

Condensing Osteitis

In a low grade infection, or when the resistance of the host is good, more and more bone deposition takes place in the existing marrow spaces. This gives rise to a uniform radiopaque shadow devoid of any marrow spaces. This radiopacity surrounds the radiolucency around the root apex. Since this condition shows condensation of bone around the root apex, it is called as condensing osteitis or sclerosing osteitis (Fig. 6.16).

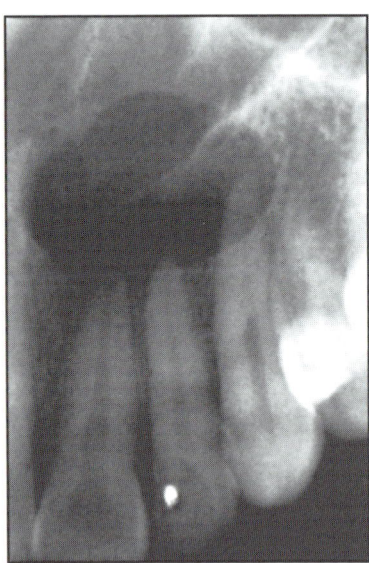

Fig. 6.13: Radiograph showing a radicular cyst.

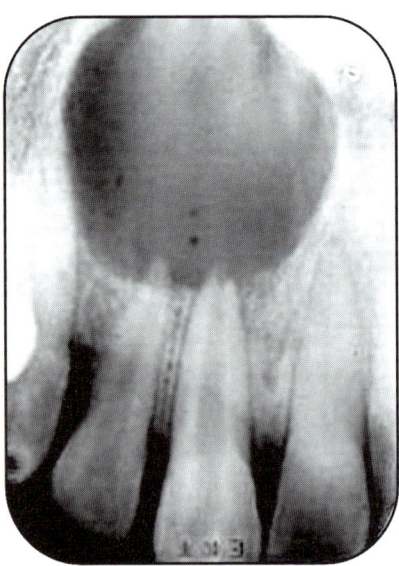

Fig. 6.14: Radiograph showing a radicular cyst. Note the open apex with central incisor which is the offending tooth.

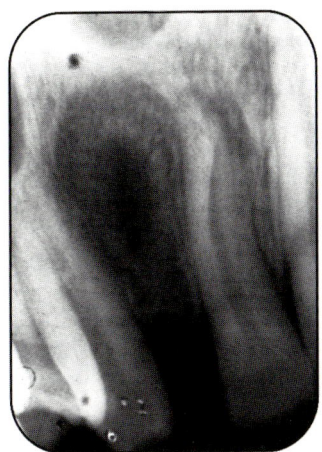

Fig. 6.15: Radiograph showing a periapical healing scar.

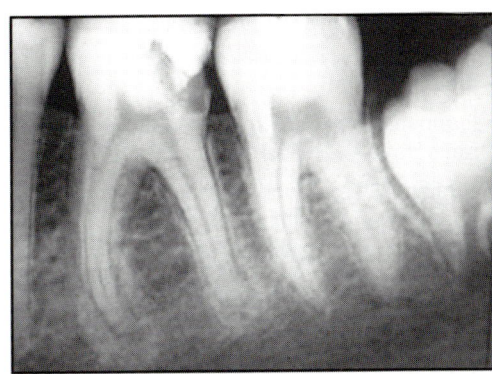

Fig. 6.16: Radiograph showing condensing osteitis in the periapical region of first molar.

DD: Osteosclerosis – It is seen in the bone as a small focal opacity in the vicinity of the tooth which is asymptomatic, whereas condensing osteitis is seen in the peri apex of a non-vital or an infected tooth. Some authors believe that osteosclerosis is nothing, but over retained deciduous root piece.

Periapical Cemental Dysplasia (PCD)/Osteofibrosis/Cementoma

This condition is frequently seen in the mandibular anterior region and is common in females of the age group of 35–40 years. More teeth than one are involved at a time and all the teeth are vital.

Stages in PCD

1. **Stage of initiation:** The periapical bone is converted into fibrous tissue and as a result, periapical radiolucency appears which can be confused with a periapical granuloma. But unlike a granuloma, the tooth is vital and lamina dura may be intact.

2. **Intermediate stage:** Deposition of bone/cementum takes place within the radiolucent zone so that the lesion appears radiolucent with radiopaque centre or as multiple areas of radiopacities (Fig. 6.17).

3. **Maturation stage:** During this stage, the entire fibrous tissue is converted into bone or cementum giving rise to a uniform radiopacity without any clear cut trabeculae. This radiopacity may have a radiolucent halo around it.

Condensing osteitis	PA cemental dysplasia
Associated with a non vital/infected tooth.	Associated with a vital tooth.
Trabeculae can be visualized within the radiopacity.	Trabeculae are not seen within the radiopacity.
It appears well demarcated on the radiograph.	It appears as a diffuse radiolucency on the radiograph.
Radiopacity surrounds a radiolucency and merges with the adjacent bone.	Radiopacity is surrounded by a radiolucent halo.

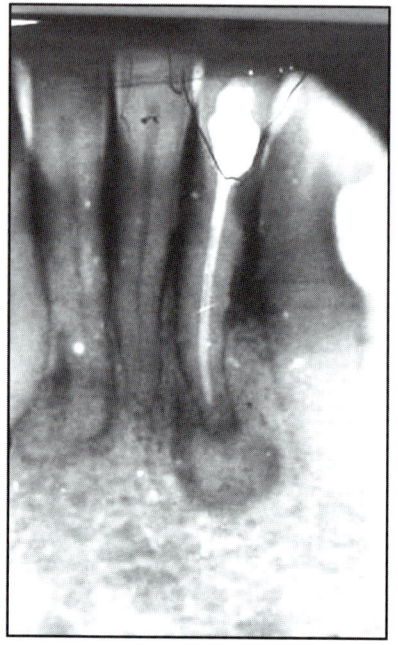

Fig. 6.17: Radiograph showing periapical cemental dysplasia in a mixed stage.

SUGGESTED READING AND REFERENCES

1. Oral Radiology—Principles and Interpretation: White and Pharoah, 5th edition.
2. Essentials of Dental Radiography and Radiology—Eric Whaites, 3rd edition.
3. The Clinical Approach to Radiographic Diagnosis—DCNA, Jan 1994.

CHAPTER 7

Periodontal Diseases

Periodontal disease collectively refers to several related disorders affecting the periodontium such as gingivitis, periodontitis, ANUG, etc. Based upon the extent of involvement and severity of the disease, it may be further classified as localized/generalized, acute/chronic.

Radiographs play a vital role in diagnosis and management of periodontal disease. They provide information regarding the amount of bone support present, type of bone loss that has occurred, width of the periodontal ligament space, presence of etiological factors like calculus, proximal overhangs, etc. Radiographs, however, have certain limitations and are complimentary to clinical examination.

LIMITATIONS OF RADIOGRAPHY

1. Acute conditions like ANUG or gingivitis cannot be seen on the radiograph.
2. Early periodontal changes cannot be seen. At least 30% of calcium must be removed from the tissues to make the changes apparent on the radiograph.
3. Bony defects on the buccal and lingual aspect of teeth cannot be seen on the radiographs.
4. Even after successfully treating the disease, the radiographs continue to show the bone loss.
5. Calculus may not be always seen on the radiograph.
6. Furcation areas may not be seen clearly on the radiographs.

In a normal young individual, the alveolar crest is at the level of the CEJ. The tip of the crest is sharp and pointed in the anterior region, while it is flat in the posterior region, making a sharp angle with the lamina dura of the teeth (Fig. 7.1).

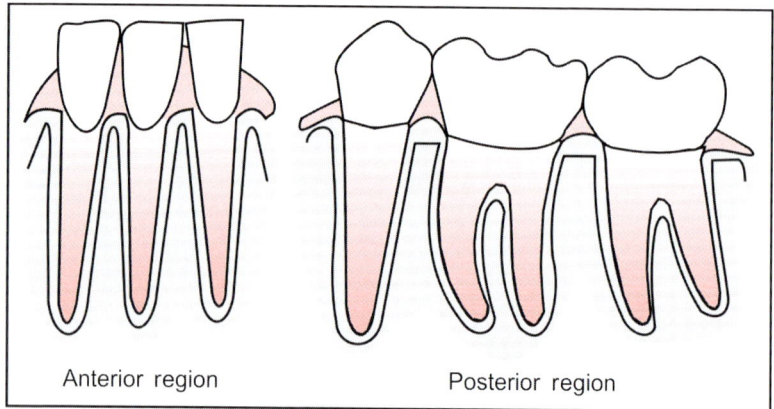

Fig. 7.1: Normal periodontal bone levels in the anterior and posterior regions.

Radiographic Findings in Periodontal Disease

In early periodontal disease, the crestal bone undergoes resorption and blunting off the tip is noticed in the anterior region. In the posterior region, the sharp angle formed by the crest of the ridge and the lamina dura becomes rounded off.

Further Loss of Bone May Follow Two Patterns

(i) *Horizontal bone loss:* It is manifested as apical migration of the crest, but the crest still remains parallel to the occlusal plane. Horizontal bone loss may be mild, moderate or severe.

(a) Mild bone loss refers to bone loss up to 1 mm from the CEJ.

(b) Moderate bone loss refers to bone loss more than 1 mm from the CEJ, up to the mid point of the roots or to the level of furcation in the posterior teeth.

(c) Severe bone loss extends beyond the mid root region and is often accompanied by furcation involvement.

(ii) *Vertical bone loss:* It refers to a pattern of bone loss in which the tip of the alveolar crest remains at the CEJ, but a defect is seen along the root surface (Figs 7.2, 7.3a and 7.3b).

Vertical bone loss may be divided into two main types

(a) *Interproximal crater:* These are two walled trough like defects that form at the crest of the interdental bone between the adjacent teeth (Figs 7.4a and b).

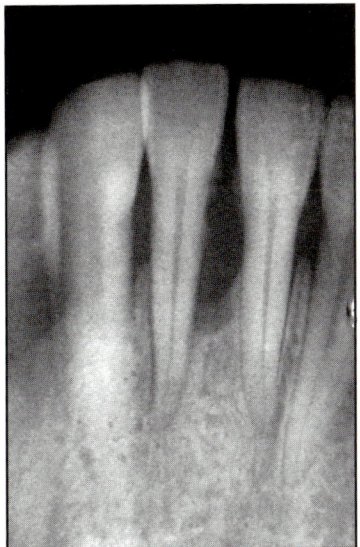

Fig. 7.2: Radiograph showing vertical bone loss with central incisor.

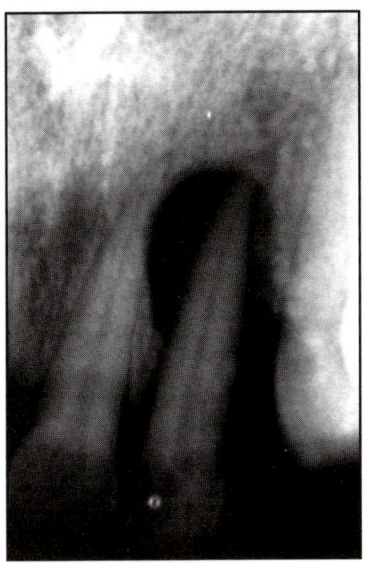

Fig. 7.3a: Radiograph showing vertical bone loss.

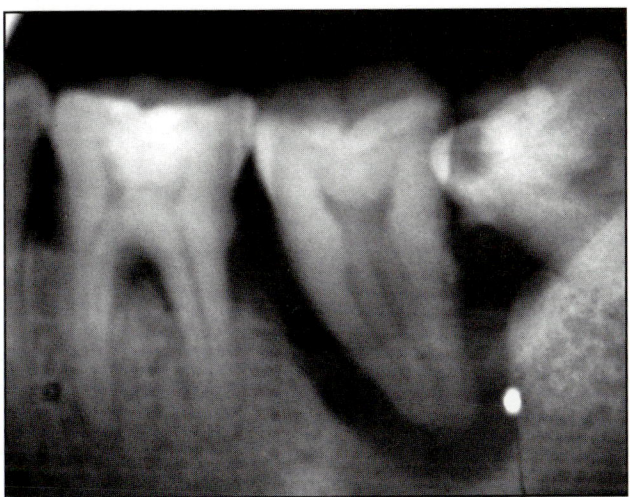

Fig. 7.3b: Radiograph showing extensive periodontal bone loss with second molar resulting in a floating tooth appearance.

(b) *Intrabony defects:* These are vertical deformities that extend apically from the crest of the bone along the root surface. Intrabony defects can be further categorized into:

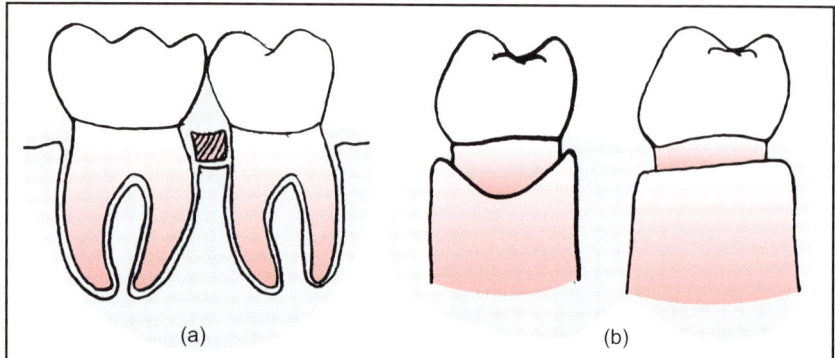

Figs 7.4a and b: (a) An interproximal crater, (b) An interproximal crater (left) and normal bone (right).

- Three-walled defect which are surrounded by three walls, i.e. when both the buccal and lingual walls are intact (Fig. 7.5).
- Two-walled defect when one of the walls has been resorbed.
- One-walled defect when one or both the buccal and lingual plates have been lost (Fig. 7.6).

Often it may be difficult to demonstrate the exact nature of these defects on a radiograph. Clinical examination, probing and surgical methods may be more useful in such cases. A radiograph made after inserting a GP point into the pocket will give a clear idea of the depth of the defect (Fig. 7.7).

Buccolingual Bone Loss

There are three radiographic findings associated with buccal/lingual bone loss as quoted by H.M. Worth.

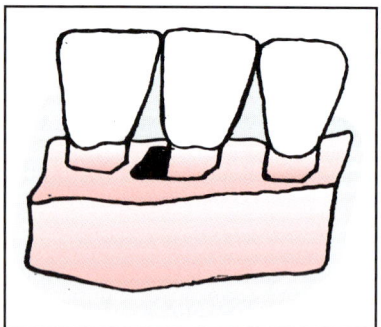

Fig. 7.5: Three-walled bony defect.

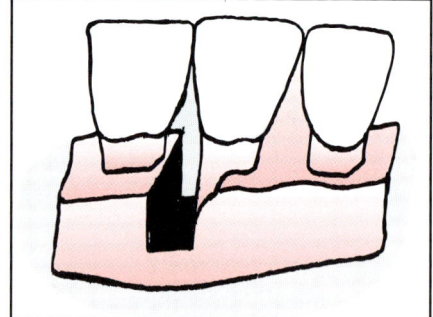

Fig. 7.6: One-walled defect in the bone.

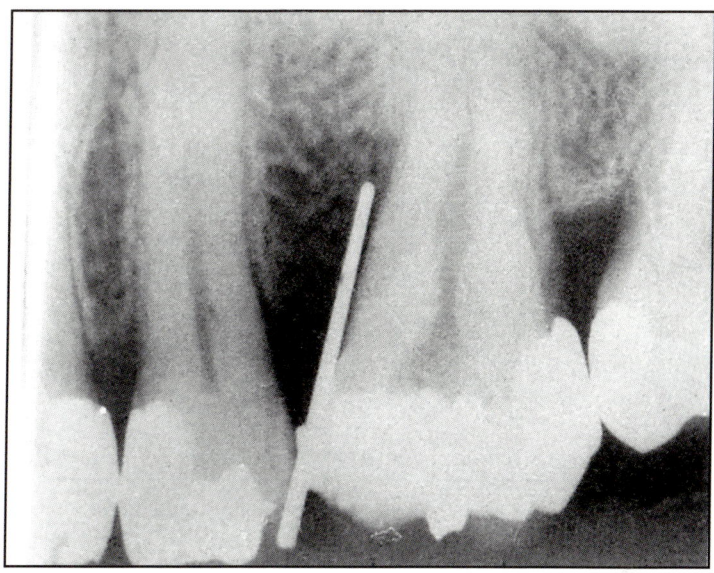

Fig. 7.7: Radiograph made with a GP point inserted in the pocket shows the depth of the defect.

(i) Two distinct borders of the alveolar crest can be traced on the shadow of the tooth (Fig. 7.8a).

(ii) A part of the shadow of the root is seen more clearly than the deeper portions and a white line can be seen on the root representing the crest of the residual ridge (Fig. 7.8b).

(iii) Alveolar recession may involve only a part of the plate (buccal or lingual) so that a portion of the width of the root is involved. This is seen as a 'J' shaped radiolucency on the root surface through which the roots are seen more clearly (Fig. 7.8c).

Alveolar Dehiscence

It is an extensive dehiscence of the buccal or lingual cortical plate resulting in exposure of the root.

Furcation Involvement

In the early stages, furcation involvement may not be seen on the radiographs because the roots may superimpose over the defect. As more and more bone is lost from the inter radicular region, the defect becomes apparent as a radiolucency in the furcation.

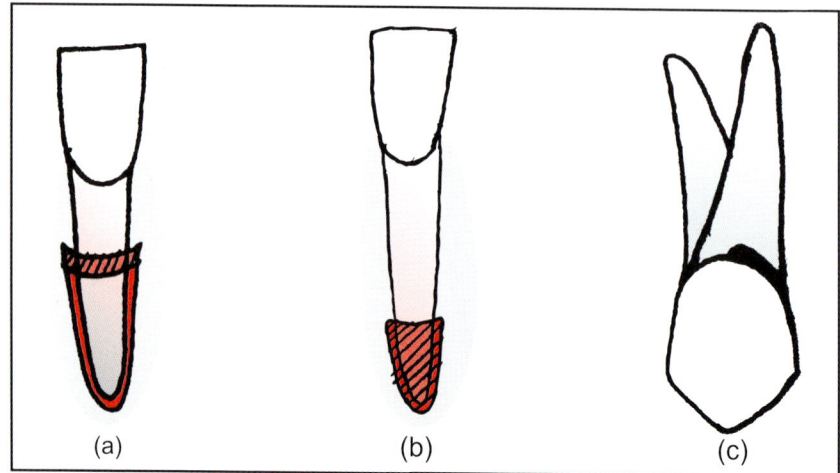

Fig. 7.8: Radiographic appearance of buccolingual bone loss.

Occlusal Trauma

It is the imbalance between the functional forces applied on the tooth and the ability of the periodontium to withstand these forces. Clinically, the teeth show occlusal facets, are sensitive to percussion and may exhibit mobility.

Radiographic changes – Resorption of the alveolar bone takes place. The resorption is more marked in the coronal and apical region, thereby giving rise to hourglass shape widening of the periodontal ligament space. The tooth may show hypercementosis, root resorption, or root fracture.

Periodontal Abscess

Periodontal abscess occurs as a part of chronic periodontitis or due to food impaction in a pocket which gets occluded and present as swelling and pain. Periodontal abscess has to be differentiated from periapical abscess clinically and radiographically.

Juvenile Periodontitis

It is a severe type of periodontitis affecting young individuals resulting in early bone loss. The bone loss is disproportionate to the amount of local factors. The most frequently affected teeth are the incisors and first permanent molars. The radiographic appearance is of a vertical, angular or arc-shaped bone loss around the affected teeth (Fig. 7.9).

Periapical abscess	Periodontal abscess
It is associated with a non-vital tooth.	It is associated with a vital tooth.
The lesion is located at the apex.	The lesion is located on the lateral aspect of the root.
Pain occurs on vertical percussion.	Pain occurs on lateral percussion.
Carious, discoloured or fractured tooth is present.	A deep periodontal pocket is seen with the lesion.
Radiographically, discontinuity of lamina dura and diffuse periapical radiolucency is seen.	Radiographically, excessive periodontal bone loss is seen associated with a diffuse radiolucency.

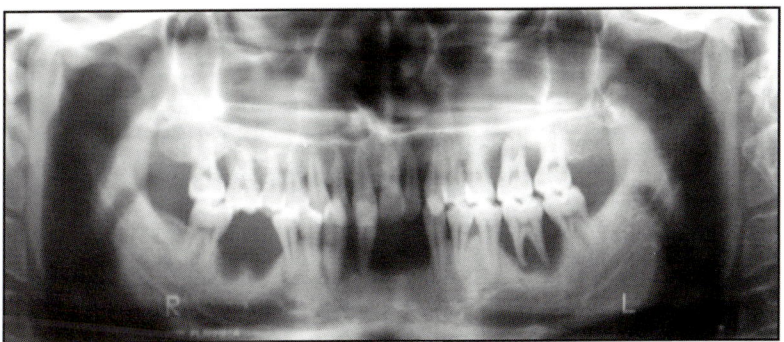

Fig. 7.9: OPG showing typical arc-shaped bone loss in the first molars in juvenile periodontitis.

SUGGESTED READING AND REFERENCES

1. Oral Radiology. Principles and Interpretation: White and Pharoah, 5th edition.
2. Essentials of Dental Radiography and Radiology. Eric Whaites, 3rd edition.
3. The Clinical Approach to Radiographic Diagnosis. DCNA Jan 1994.
4. Principles and Practice of Oral Radiographic Interpretations. H.M. Worth.

Notes

CHAPTER 8

Osteomyelitis

Osteomyelitis is an inflammatory disease of the bone involving the spongiosa and compact cortical plates. Osteomyelitis is seen commonly in the mandible as it has less blood supply and dense cortical plates. Maxilla has more marrow spaces, hence osteomyelitis of hematogenous origin is more common in the maxilla.

Etiology

1. The most important cause of osteomyelitis of the jaws is sequelae of dental caries and periapical infection. Fractures of the teeth can also result into osteomyelitis.
2. Fracture of the jaws following trauma can lead to osteomyelitis.
3. Exanthematous fever like scarlet fever, etc.
4. Systemic infections like tuberculosis and syphilis.
5. Metal poisoning.
6. Any condition that results in avascular bone is more prone to undergo osteomyelitis, e.g. osteoradionecrosis, Paget's disease, osteopetrosis, fluorosis.
7. Herpes zoster infection if severe and left untreated is reported to be associated with exfoliation of teeth and osteomyelitis.

Pathogenesis

(i) Virulent organisms reach the depth of the bone as a result of the above mentioned causes and set up an inflammatory reaction. In the normal course, the pus formed is either drained surgically or discharged through a sinus tract.

(ii) In osteomyelitis, the infection spreads rapidly through the bone and reaches the cortex. It then perforates the cortex and reaches the under surface of the periosteum.

(iii) At this stage, it starts spreading sub periosteally over the surface of the bone.

(iv) Pus now enters the depth of the bone from a different site through the Volkmann's canals.

(v) As a result of entry of pus into the Volkmann's canals, the blood vessels in the canal shows stasis of blood followed by thrombosis and embolism.

(vi) Due to thrombosis, the part of the bone in that area undergoes necrosis and forms the sequestrum. Thus in osteomyelitis, the infection spreads not only within the bone, but also sub periosteally and gives rise to involvement of a large part of the bone.

(vii) The sequestra may exfoliate or may be removed surgically.

(viii) Periosteum is stimulated in the involved region to form new bone called the involucrum. The function of the involucrum is to join the two living fragments of the bone and maintain the integrity of the bone.

(ix) Involucrum formation is greater in young individuals due to higher osteogenic potential of the bone.

(x) On the surface of the involucrum, small orifices are formed called cloacae through which the pus continuously oozes out as it communicates with the focus of infection.

(xi) After the removal of sequestrum, resorption of involucrum takes place and the bone may recover its original shape.

Clinical Features of Osteomyelitis

(a) The patient usually gives a history of painful tooth, trauma or fracture of the jaws.

(b) Severe pain, swelling, and redness are usually the presenting symptoms.

(c) Multiple discharging sinuses may be present intraorally or on the facial skin.

(d) Fever and lymphadenopathy also may be present.

(e) Reflex spasm of the muscles may lead to trismus.

(f) Paresthesia of the lip may be present if the inferior alveolar nerve is affected.

(g) In the oral cavity, bare bone may be seen without the mucosal covering, which is painful.

(h) Predisposing factors for osteomyelitis like old age, anemia, sickle cell anemia, history of radiotherapy, tuberculosis, etc. may be present in most cases.

Radiographic Features

The various radiographic features of osteomyelitis are:

1. In the acute stage, since 30% of calcium is not removed from the bone, radiographic changes may not be apparent. As the condition becomes more chronic, the trabeculae become thinner and sometimes destroyed giving rise to a diffuse irregular radiolucency.

2. Within this radiolucency, sequestrum appears as areas of radiopacity. The sequestra appear more radiopaque because:
   (i) Condensation of bone takes place before the blood supply is cut off.
   (ii) Since the blood supply is cut off, no calcium is being removed or added as opposed to normal bone.
   (iii) Optical illusion: The appearance of the sequestrum as a dense radiopaque mass may be an optical illusion against the surrounding areas which appear more radiolucent due to the infectious process.

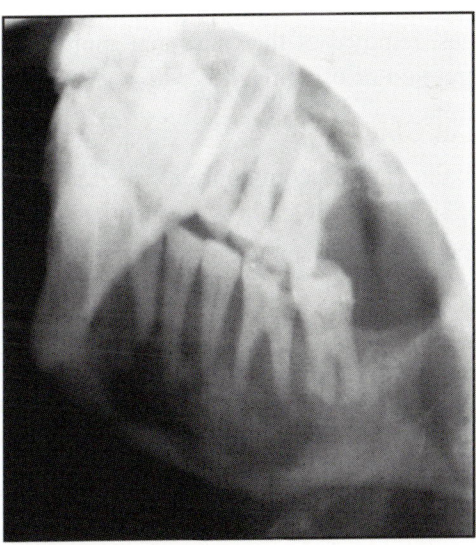

Fig 8.1: Lateral oblique view showing moth-eaten appearance of the mandible with sequestrum and floating tooth.

3. The sequestrae may be single, multiple, small or large.

4. Islands of normal bone can be seen surrounding the sequestrum.

5. The lamina dura of the teeth in the affected area is missing.

6. When osteomyelitis affects children, the cortical outline of the developing follicles become inconspicuous.

7. The deposition of new bone/involucrum is seen as a dull grey shadow parallel to the lower border of the mandible on a lateral oblique view or an OPG. It may also be seen as a dull grey shadow parallel to the buccal/lingual cortices of the jaws on a true occlusal view.

8. Overall radiographic appearance of osteomyelitis is described as a *'moth-eaten'* (Fig. 8.1). The teeth in the vicinity may loose bone support and present as a *'floating tooth appearance'* (Fig. 8.1).

Limitations of Radiographs in the Diagnosis of Osteomyelitis

(a) Acute changes are not visualized on the radiographs.

(b) The periosteum is not visualized on the radiograph unless new bone formation has taken place.

Treatment of Osteomyelitis

In the acute stages, removal of the cause and appropriate antibiotics can prevent the progression of osteomyelitis.

Osteomyelitis in Children

1. The maxilla is more commonly affected in children because the mode of spread of infection is through haematogenous route.

2. Radiographic changes may not be apparent because there are many developing teeth within the jaws and very few trabeculae are visible on the radiograph.

3. Occasionally, disappearance of the cortical lining of the follicle may be the only radiographic sign of osteomyelitis in children.

4. Teeth may appear to have been moved within the bone.

5. Sequestration is similar to that of adults but may not be visible on the radiographs.

6. Osteogenic potential of bone is more in children and hence periosteal reaction is marked in children.

Garre's Osteomyelitis

Garre's osteomyelitis is a condition seen in young individuals when the offending infection is mild. It may give rise to spindle-shaped enlargement of mandible. Radiographically, it appears as diffuse sclerosis of the bone. On an occlusal view, alternate laminations of radiopaque and radiolucent bands are seen. This is referred to as an *onion skin appearance*. (Figs 8.2 and 8.3).

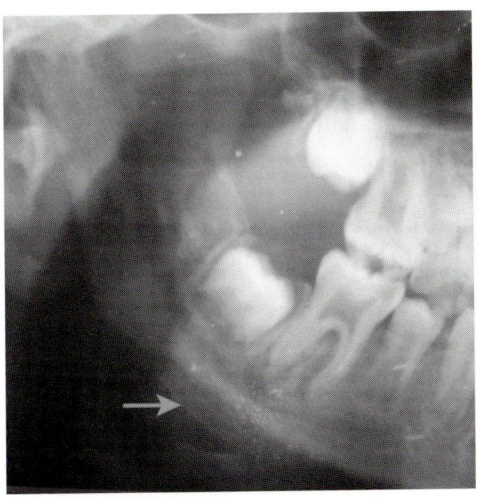

Fig. 8.2: Radiograph showing periosteal reaction at the lower border of the mandible (arrow).

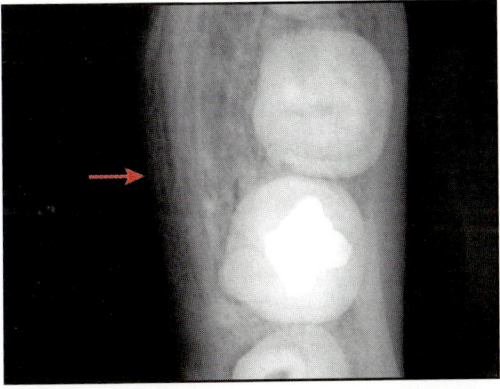

Fig. 8.3: Occlusal view showing periosteal reaction along the buccal cortical plate (arrow).

Diffuse Sclerosing Osteomyelitis

When a sub virulent infection affects a patient with a good general resistance, more and more deposition of bone takes place within the bone marrow. This gives rise to large areas of diffuse radiopacity in the jaws. Sometimes during periods of acute exacerbation, areas of radiolucency may be seen. Scintigraphy with technetium pertechnetate[99] shows an area of greater uptake of the radio tracer in the area of bone formation.

Tuberculosis and syphilis may involve the bone, but from the radiographic finding alone, it is difficult to arrive at any specific diagnosis. The lesion of syphilis which involves the bone is called gumma, which may give rise to perforation of the palate. Some believe that the sequestrae formed in syphilis are small and may be absorbed in the blood stream.

Osteoradionecrosis

This is a complication resulting in bones which have received high doses of therapeutic radiation. This condition has been discussed in chapter 2.

SUGGESTED READING AND REFERENCES

1. Oral Radiology—Principles and Interpretation: White & Pharoah—5th edition.
2. Principles and Practice of Oral Radiographic Interpretations—H.M. Worth.
3. Oral and Maxillofacial Infections—Topazian and Goldberg.

9

Cysts of the Jaws

Definition

According to *Kramer*, a cyst may be defined as a pathological cavity containing fluid, semi fluid or gaseous contents, which may or may not be lined by epithelium and is not formed by accumulation of pus.

Classification of Cyst (By Shear)

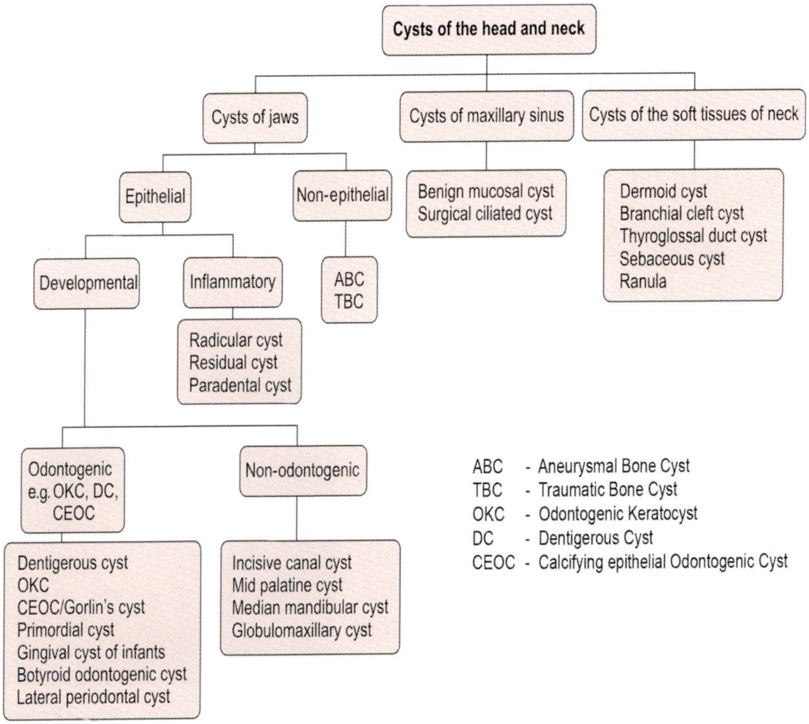

Cysts of the head and neck

- Cysts of jaws
  - Epithelial
    - Developmental
      - Odontogenic e.g. OKC, DC, CEOC
        - Dentigerous cyst
        - OKC
        - CEOC/Gorlin's cyst
        - Primordial cyst
        - Gingival cyst of infants
        - Botyroid odontogenic cyst
        - Lateral periodontal cyst
      - Non-odontogenic
        - Incisive canal cyst
        - Mid palatine cyst
        - Median mandibular cyst
        - Globulomaxillary cyst
    - Inflammatory
      - Radicular cyst
      - Residual cyst
      - Paradental cyst
  - Non-epithelial
    - ABC
    - TBC
- Cysts of maxillary sinus
  - Benign mucosal cyst
  - Surgical ciliated cyst
- Cysts of the soft tissues of neck
  - Dermoid cyst
  - Branchial cleft cyst
  - Thyroglossal duct cyst
  - Sebaceous cyst
  - Ranula

ABC - Aneurysmal Bone Cyst
TBC - Traumatic Bone Cyst
OKC - Odontogenic Keratocyst
DC - Dentigerous Cyst
CEOC - Calcifying epithelial Odontogenic Cyst

Characteristic Features of Cyst

1. *Slow growth:* Cyst shows a very slow growth allowing sufficient time for the body to wall it off.

2. *Expansion of bone:* As the cyst grows in size due to increased osmotic and hydrostatic pressure or due to epithelial growth, it causes expansion of bone.

3. *Growth by expansion:* As the cyst expands, more and more bone is resorbed as the cyst reaches the periosteum. At this stage, osteoblastic layer is stimulated to lay down new bone which is again resorbed by the growing cyst. This is once again followed by new bone formation. This phenomenon is called growth by expansion (Fig. 9.1).

4. Disfigurement of face results due to swelling.

5. *Egg shell crackling:* The cortex of the bone becomes extremely thin due to expansion and digital pressure gives rise to a egg shell cracking sensation.

6. *Perforation:* At times the cyst grows faster than the subperiosteal bone deposition. This gives rise to destruction of the bone and formation of a window through which the cystic contents may protrude and fluctuation may be elicited. The cyst which extends into the soft tissues may be traumatized and secondarily infected giving rise to pain and swelling.

7. *Paresthesia:* The growing cyst may cause a pressure on the neurovascular bundle giving rise to paresthesia and numbness/tingling sensation. This is called as ***Vincent's sign***.

8. *Displacement of anatomical landmarks:* Cyst which may lie close to the mandibular canal or the maxillary sinus can cause displacement of these anatomic structures, but no destruction is seen. The floor of the maxillary

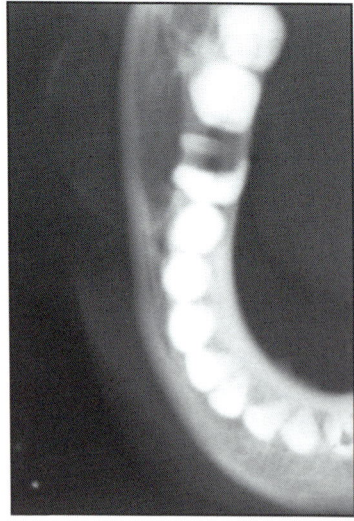

Fig. 9.1: Occlusal view showing expansion of bone caused by a cyst.

sinus which is seen as a convexity pointing downwards undergoes a change, so that the floor becomes concave but remains traceable without any break. Malignant conditions on the other hand give rise to destruction and break in the continuity of the floor of sinus.

RADICULAR CYST

A radicular cyst is one which is associated with the apex of a deeply carious and /or a non-vital tooth.

Pathogenesis

1. The source of epithelium in this cyst is from the cell rests of Malassez, Hertwig's epithelial root sheath, dental lamina, the oral epithelium or the lining of the maxillary sinus.

2. The cyst forms as a result of degeneration of the epithelial cells within the granuloma or proliferation of epithelial cells around the abscess cavity.

Radiographic Features

(i) The cyst appears as a round or oval-shaped radiolucency with smooth round continuous and corticated margins. The borders of the cyst may be defined as sclerotic or hyperostotic (Figs 9.2 and 6.14).

(ii) The lamina dura around the affected tooth is discontinuous and is continuous with the cortex of the cyst.

(iii) In case of a large radiolucent lesion appearing to involve the periapical area of multiple teeth, the offending tooth can be identified by:

(a) a large and wide root canal because the odontoblasts become inactive in a non-vital tooth.

(b) a wide apical foramen.

(c) evidence of root resorption, i.e. a blunt apex.

(iv) Sometimes the cyst may grow so rapidly than the sub periosteal reaction that it may give rise to perforation in the bone (Fig. 9.3). This is called window formation and appears on the radiograph as an area of increased radiolucency within the cystic radiolucency due to the absence of the bony wall.

(v) Radiolucency around the root apex of a non-vital tooth must be differentiated from an apical scar or a surgical defect.

RESIDUAL CYST

A residual cyst is one which remains even after the extraction of the offending tooth. It appears on the radiograph as a well-defined radiolucent lesion in the mandible or maxilla (Fig. 9.4). Quite often, the lamina dura of the offending tooth does not undergo complete decalcification and remains continuous with the cystic radiolucency.

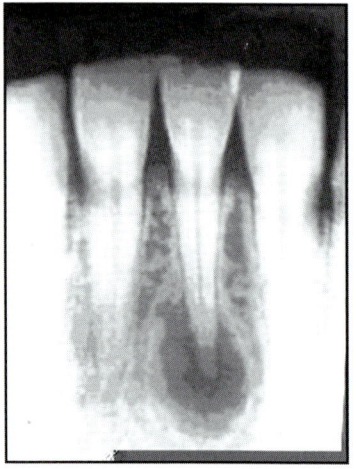

Fig. 9.2: Radiograph showing a radicular cyst.

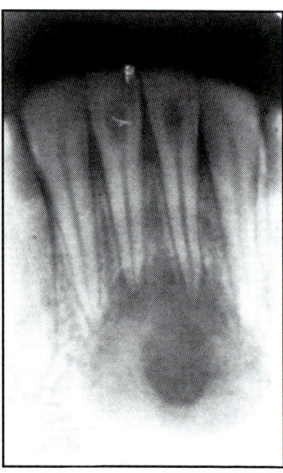

Fig. 9.3: Radiograph showing a radicular cyst causing perforation of bone and window formation.

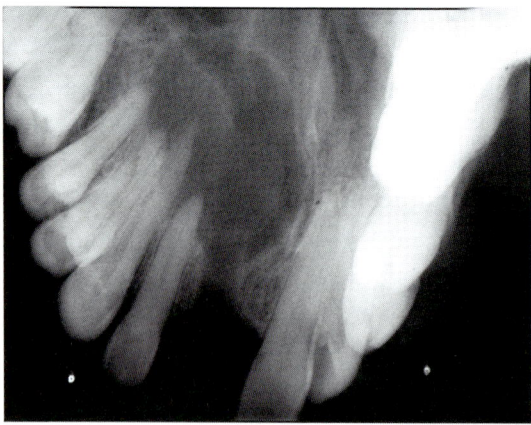

Fig. 9.4: Radiograph showing a residual cyst in the maxilla.

PRIMORDIAL CYST

According to Robinson, a primordial cyst is one which forms from the degeneration of the stellate reticulum of the enamel organ before the formation of hard tissues.

It is derived from the odontogenic primordium and occurs in place of a missing tooth. At times when all the teeth are present, primordial cyst may be derived from the follicle of a supernumerary tooth.

Primordial cysts are frequently seen in the younger age group and show rapid growth through the cancellous bone without causing much expansion of bone.

Aspiration of a primordial cyst yields a thick, granular, yellowish material instead of a straw coloured fluid. The yellowish colour may be due to the presence of keratin in the lumen of the cyst.

Types of Primordial Cysts

1. Replacemental type which forms in place of a missing tooth.
2. Collateral type which forms between the two roots resembling a lateral periodontal cyst.
3. Envelopmental type that surrounds the crown of an unerupted tooth.
4. Extraneous type which is found in the ramus.

Radiographic Appearance

(i) The lesion appears as a large well-defined radiolucency having a smooth round corticated border.

(ii) Primordial cysts occur frequently in the ramus, where due to the strong attachment of masseter to the middle part of the ramus, it does not expand giving rise to the appearance of a septum inside the lesion.

(iii) Also due to the presence of a thick cortex laterally, buccal expansion is not as prominent as lingual expansion.

D.D.—Benign tumors: They are usually multilocular and a break or notch in the cortex may be seen. Septa and trabeculae are also present frequently within a benign tumor.

DENTIGEROUS CYST

1. A dentigerous cyst is one which forms around the crown of a developing tooth due to accumulation of fluid between the crown and the reduced enamel epithelium.

2. Based upon the pattern of growth of the cyst and its relation to the crown, dentigerous cyst can be of three types: the central, lateral and circumferential.

3. The lesion is most commonly associated with an impacted mandibular third molar and has a strong potential to cause expansion.

4. Displacement of teeth is commonly seen and the mandibular third molars may be displaced towards the inferior cortex or high up in the ramus.

5. Radiographically dentigerous cysts are seen as peri coronal radiolucency with well-demarcated and corticated margins (Fig. 9.5).

6. Expansion of the cortices can be seen on occlusal radiographs.

7. Root resorption is also a prominent finding with dentigerous cysts.

D.D.: AOT, CEOT, ameloblastic fibroma and other pericoronal radiolucencies.

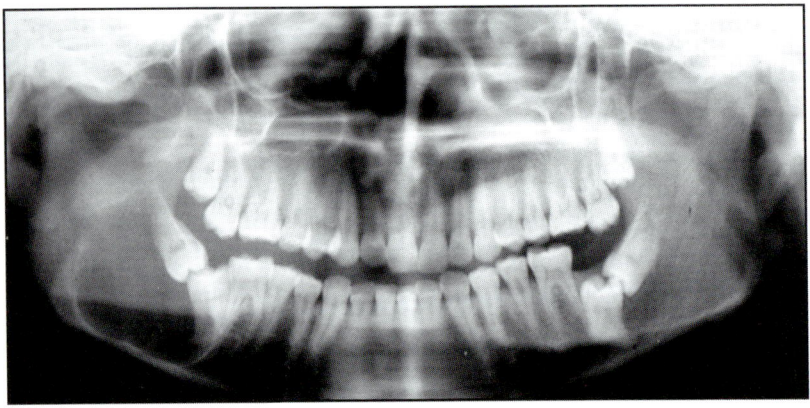

Fig. 9.5: OPG showing dentigerous cyst in the right ramus.

Complications of Dentigerous Cyst

(i) It may prevent tooth eruption.

(ii) Mural ameloblastomas may arise from the lining of the cyst.

(iii) Mucoepidermoid carcinomas may arise from the lining of the cyst.

Since the maxillary sinus appears radiolucent with a corticated outline, it resembles a cyst and must therefore be differentiated.

Cyst	Maxillary sinus
Cyst contains fluid and hence it appears less radiolucent.	Maxillary sinus contains air and hence appears more radiolucent.
The corticated outline of the cyst has convexity pointing upwards.	The corticated outline of the sinus has convexity pointing downwards.
The cortical outline is continuous with the follicle of the teeth.	It appears as a separate radiolucency not continuous with the crown.
The margins are smooth, round, corticated and continuous.	The margins are thicker and serrated.
Vascular channels are not seen on the walls of a cyst.	Vascular channels may be seen on the walls of the sinus.
A cyst usually causes expansion.	Expansion is not a feature with sinus.

ODONTOGENIC KERATOCYST

1. It is an odontogenic epithelial cyst that arises from the dental lamina or the basal cells of the oral epithelium.

2. The epithelial lining of the cyst is thin and made up of 5–7 layers of cells with a thick corrugated layer of keratin lining the lumen. Budlike projections may be given out by the epithelium which gives rise to daughter cyst in the connective tissue wall. Presence of such daughter cyst results in a high rate of recurrence.

3. The lumen of the cyst also contains keratin flecks and aspiration may yield thick granular material instead of a straw colored fluid.

4. The lesion is often very aggressive and shows rapid growth.

5. Radiographically, the lesion appears as a large multilocular radiolucency with well-corticated margins, often associated with an impacted tooth (Fig. 9.6).

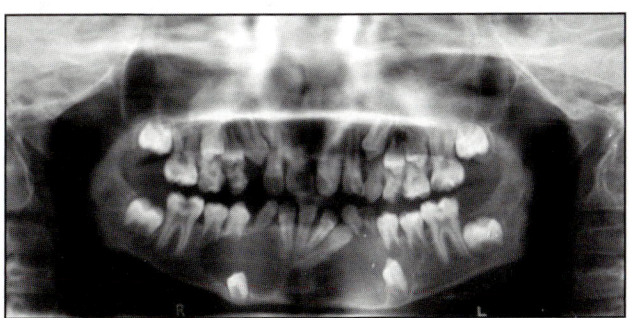

Fig. 9.6: Multiple OKCs in a patient with Gorlin-Goltz syndrome.

6. In the anterior region, the lesion may cross the midline.
7. OKC has a high recurrence rate after treatment.

Gorlin-Goltz Syndrome/Nevoid Basal Cell Carcinoma Syndrome

It is an autosomal dominant condition in which the patient may present with multiple OKCs in the jaws. Other findings associated with this syndrome include:

(i) Multiple basal cell carcinomas of the skin

(ii) Bifid rib

(iii) Frontal bossing

(iv) Hypertelorism

(v) Depressed nose bridge

(vi) Calcification of falx cerebri

(vii) Palmar plantar pits

D.D. - OKC must be differentiated from benign tumors such as ameloblastoma, giant cell granuloma. While cysts usually show buccal expansion, tumors may exhibit buccolingual expansion.

Causes of High Recurrence Rate of OKC

(a) Presence of *daughter cysts* in the connective tissue wall.

(b) Thin lining of the cyst which makes complete enucleation of the lesion very difficult.

(c) The scalloped margins of the lesion resulting due to differential growth of the lesion also make complete removal of the lining very difficult.

(d) Association with Gorlin-Goltz syndrome increases the chances of recurrence.

LATERAL PERIODONTAL CYST

1. The lateral periodontal cyst arises in the periodontium and is located in the interproximal bone between the apex and the alveolar crest.

2. The cells lining the lateral periodontal cyst may resemble the clear cells of the dental lamina.

3. The cyst may be located bucally or lingually.

4. Radiographically, the cyst may appear as a round or oval-shaped radiolucency in between the roots of the premolars (Fig. 9.7).

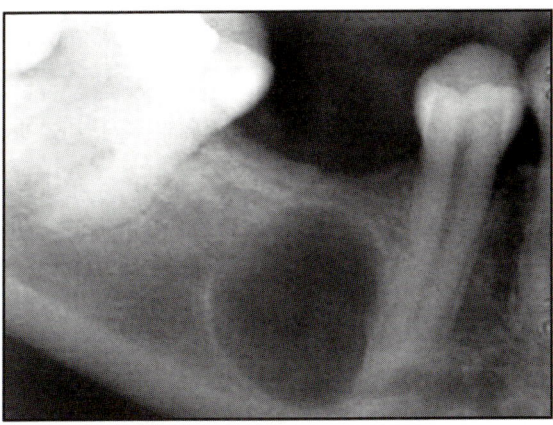

Fig. 9.7: Radiograph showing a lateral periodontal cyst.

GLOBULOMAXILLARY CYST

1. The globulomaxillary cyst was believed to be a fissural cyst arising from the epithelium entrapped between the globular process of the maxilla and the maxillary process. But now it is believed that this cyst is not a fissural cyst, but a primordial cyst arising in the globulo-maxillary area.

2. Clinically, it presents as a slow growing enlargement between the maxillary lateral incisors and the canine. This results in displacement of the roots of these teeth and the contact point moves more incisally.

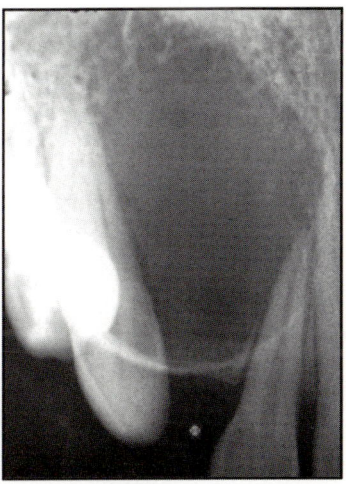

3. The adjacent teeth are vital.

4. Radiographically, the lesion appears as an inverted pear-shaped radiolucency with the apex pointing towards the inter dental crest. The radiolucency is surrounded by a corticated border (Fig. 9.8).

5. Lamina dura of the teeth in the vicinity are intact.

Fig. 9.8: IOPA view showing a globulo-maxillary cyst between the canine and lateral incisor.

Radicular cyst	Globulo-maxillary cyst
The associated teeth are non-vital.	The associated teeth are vital.
Lamina dura is discontinuous apically, but continuous with the cortex of the cyst.	Lamina dura is continuous apically.
The lesion occupies the space around the apex of the tooth.	The lesion occupies the space lateral to the root surface.

D.D.: Radicular cyst

CALCIFYING EPITHELIAL ODONTOGENIC CYST (CEOC)/ GORLIN'S CYST

1. It is an uncommon, slowly growing benign entity. The lesion shows many characteristics of a tumor and hence placed between a cyst and the tumor.
2. CEOC usually occurs in younger age group in the region anterior to the first molars in the maxilla and mandible.
3. Radiographically, the lesion appears as a radiolucency which may be unilocular or multilocular.
4. Inside the lumen of the lesion, areas of calcification are seen as radiopaque specks.
5. The cyst may also cause resorption or perforation of the cortex.

D.D.: Cystic odontome, AOT, Ossifying fibroma.

Treatment: Surgical enucleation.

MEDIAN MANDIBULAR CYST

1. This cyst occurs between the roots of mandibular central incisors causing displacement of the roots.
2. The teeth are however vital.
3. Radiographically, it is seen as round or ovoid radiolucency with corticated margins, but the lamina dura is intact.

MEDIAN PALATINE CYST/ANTERIOR PALATINE CYST/ ANTERIOR ALVEOLAR CYST

1. It is believed to be a fissural cyst arising from the epithelial remnants of the cells in the line of fusion.

2. It appears on the radiographs as a well-defined heart-shaped radiolucent lesion due to the superimposition of the anterior nasal spine (Fig. 9.9).

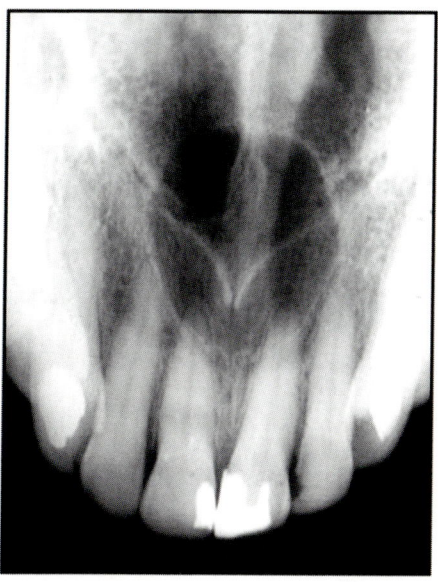

Fig. 9.9: Radiograph showing mid palatine cyst appearing as a heart-shaped radiolucency.

3. Lamina dura of these teeth are intact and the cyst appears in the mid line, bilaterally symmetrical.
4. The adjacent teeth are vital.

INCISIVE FORAMEN CYST

1. The normal incisive foramen appears on the radiograph between the two central incisors as an oval-shaped radiolucency having the largest diameter of 6 mm (Fig. 9.10).
2. When cyst formation takes place, it appears radiographically as a radiolucent lesion larger than 1 cm. The incisive foramen shows cortication on the sides, whereas the cyst appears rounded with cortication around the entire lesion (Fig. 9.10).
3. Clinically, swelling is usually present palatally, and aspiration yields fluid from which the diagnosis can be made.

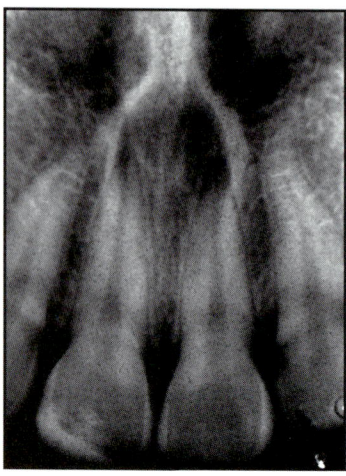

Fig. 9.10: Radiograph showing an incisive foramen cyst.

NASOPALATINE CYST

1. It develops from the nasopalatine duct which is located in the nasopalatine canal.
2. The lesion may be clinically asymptomatic or sometimes a bluish red palatal swelling may appear.
3. Numbness of the palatal mucosa may be present in the anterior region due to compression of the neurovascular bundle by the lesion.
4. Radiologically, it shows as a heart-shaped radiolucent lesion due to the superimposition of anterior nasal spine.
5. Change in the angulation causes the radiolucency to be cast away from the incisors more so since the nasopalatine canal is located closer to the tube.

NASOLABIAL CYST

1. It is located in the naso labial fold as a unilateral swelling distorting the nostril and causing fullness of the lips.
2. Swelling may be visualized in the floor of the nasal cavity.
3. At times, it may cause difficulty in breathing through the affected nostril.
4. Difficulty may be encountered while making a complete denture if the lesion fills up the labial sulcus.

5. Since the lesion is located within the soft tissues, no radiographic changes are expected. However the lesion may cause depression of the bone and cause increased radiolucency of the bone in the affected region.

6. Also it may cause posterior bowing of the floor of nasal cavity which may be seen on an occlusal radiograph.

STAFNE'S CYST/LATENT BONE CYST

1. It is a pseudo cyst caused due to depression in the lower border of the mandible to accommodate the submandibular salivary gland.

2. It appears as a semicircular radiolucency at the lower border of mandible just posterior to the point where the facial artery crosses the lower border of the mandible (Fig. 9.11).

3. It is asymptomatic and does not grow in size. Hence, it is called as a static bone cyst.

4. A sialography will confirm the presence of salivary gland tissue within the radiolucency.

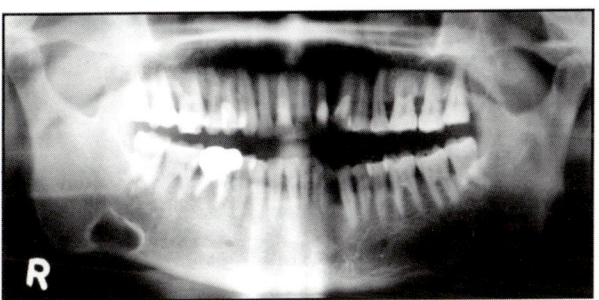

Fig. 9.11: OPG showing a Stafne's bone cyst.

TRAUMATIC BONE CYST

1. Traumatic bone cyst is common in younger individuals because they have more blood supply to the teeth and their bone is more resilient which does not fracture after trauma. Sometimes, there may also be deficiency in the clotting factors.

2. Pathogenesis: As a result of trauma, haematoma is formed within the bone, but organization of clot does not take place giving rise to a cavity within the bone. It is not a true cyst because it is devoid of any lining.

3. Clinically, there may be an asymptomatic swelling, but firm digital pressure may elicit a smarting pain.
4. Radiographically, it appears as a unilocular radiolucency with well-defined borders. The lesion protrudes between the roots and has scalloped margins (Fig. 9.12).
5. Aspiration yields a serosanguineous fluid.

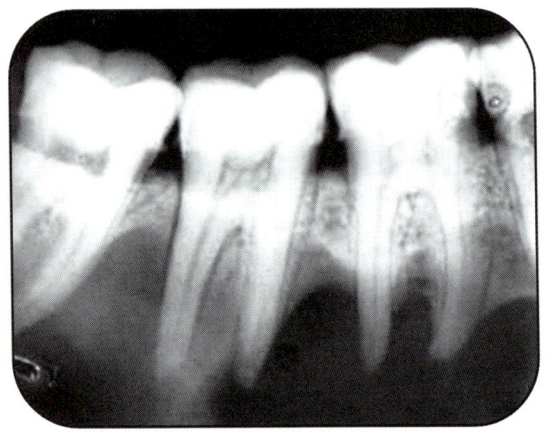

Fig. 9.12: Radiograph showing a traumatic bone cyst.

ANEURYSMAL BONE CYST (ABC)

1. It forms because of sudden venous occlusion of the arteriovenous shunt. There is dilatation of the blood vessel causing ballooning of the bone.
2. Radiographically, it is seen as a unilocular/multilocular radiolucency with well-demarcated borders. The typical radiographic appearance is called as soap bubble appearance.
3. During surgery, when the cystic cavity is opened, pooling of blood takes place and the hemorrhage is difficult to manage.
4. The cystic lumen contains friable, vascular tissue which subdivides the lumen into a number of compartments.

D.D.: Benign tumors such as ameloblastomas, myxomas must be differentiated from ABC.

BENIGN MUCOSAL CYST OF THE MAXILLARY ANTRUM

1. It is a lesion which may be unilateral or bilateral within the maxillary sinus.

2. The condition may be asymptomatic or cause a dull pain with a significant difficulty in breathing through the nostril of the affected side.

3. Post nasal discharge may be present.

4. Radiographically, a dome-shaped opaque shadow may be seen inside the sinus. The walls of the sinus appear to be intact (Fig. 9.13).

5. The superior surface of the cyst does not have a bony wall which serves to differentiate it from extrinsic cysts which have a cortical wall around them.

D.D.: Antral polyp. When an antral polyp is present, the entire mucosa of the sinus appears to be thickened.

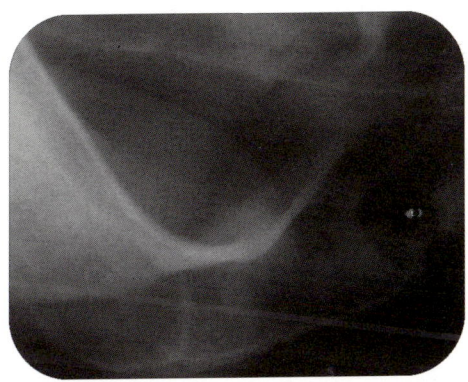

Fig. 9.13: Edentulous maxilla showing a benign mucosal cyst in the antrum.

MUCOCELE

1. It is seen as a soft blue fluctuant swelling on the lower lip. The lesion is more common on the lower lip because it is more prone to trauma.

2. When it ruptures, it gives out a sticky fluid with a salty taste.

3. A mucocele may be caused due to two reasons:

   (a) extravasation of gland secretions.

   (b) retention of mucous.

BUCCAL BIFURCATION CYST

1. It is a cyst which is derived from the epithelial remnants of the cells on the periodontal membrane of the buccal bifurcation area.

2. The common presenting feature is the delay in the eruption of the mandibular first or second molar.

3. On clinical examination, the lingual cusp tips of the unerupted molar appear to be projecting out abnormally.

4. A hard swelling may be present buccally. Pain is not a feature unless secondarily infected.

5. Radiographically, it appears as radiolucency superimposed over the roots of the first molar.

6. The involved molar is tipped with its roots lingually and the crown bucally making the occlusal surface visible on the radiograph.

7. A large cyst may cause tooth displacement and smooth expansion of the cortical plate.

SUGGESTED READING AND REFERENCES

1. Oral Radiology—Principles and Interpretation: White & Pharoah—5th edition.
2. Essentials of Dental Radiography and Radiology. Eric Whaites, 3rd edition.
3. Cysts of the Oral Region. Shear, 3rd edition.
4. Principles and Practice of Oral Radiographic Interpretations—H.M.Worth.
5. Differential Diagnosis of Oral Lesions. Wood & Goaz.
6. Panoramic Radiology-Langland.

CHAPTER 10

Odontomes and Benign Tumors

Hamartomas are tissue growths which do not have limitless proliferative capacity. They are derived from the cells naturally existing in that area, e.g. lymphangioma, hemangioma and odontomes.

Odontomes are believed to be hamartomas of dental origin which are derived from the primordial odontogenic cells during the period of tooth development and they do not grow beyond a particular limit.

CLASSIFICATION OF ODONTOME

1. Ectodermal – Enameloma
2. Mesodermal – Dentinoma
   – Cementoma
   – Benign cementoblastoma.
3. Mixed – Complex composite odontome and its cystic variety
   – Compound composite odontome and its cystic variety
   – Geminated odontome
   – Dilated odontome:
       (i) dens in dente
       (ii) root dilation
       (iii) inverted open umbrella
       (iv) fleur-de-lys

ENAMELOMA

1. It is seen as a nodule of enamel attached to the C-E junction most commonly at the furcation area of multi rooted teeth (Fig. 10.1).

2. Since it is made of enamel, it appears on the radiograph as a round radiopaque mass. It is also called as enamel pearl (Fig. 10.2).

3. If located near the gingival margin, it causes irritation and pocket formation. Hence such structures should be sliced off.

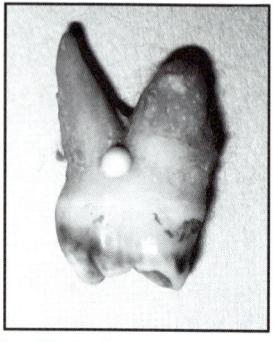

Fig. 10.1: An enameloma in a maxillary molar.

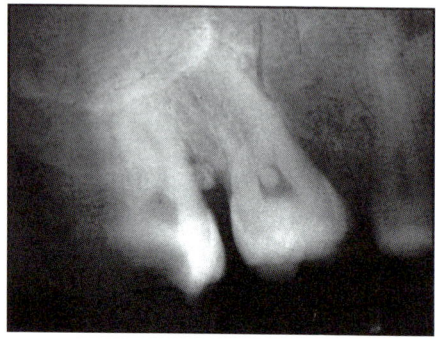

Fig. 10.2: Radiograph showing enameloma on the mesial surface of the second molar.

D/D :

(i) Calculus: Supragingival calculus is sharp and pointed and less radiopaque than enamel.

(ii) Radiopaque shadow caused due to the superimposition of two or three roots of the teeth may also appear like an enameloma. To differentiate between the two, another radiograph must be obtained with a change in the angulation. The shadow caused due to superimposition of the roots will disappear in the second radiograph. Periphery of the shadow is continuous with the periodontal ligament space of the roots.

DENTINOMA

It is a very rare tumor because it is rare that the dentine will alone form excessively without the formation of enamel. However, when dentinoma occurs it is seen as a radiopaque mass surrounded by a radiolucent line suggestive of a fibrous capsule which in turn is surrounded by a radiopaque cortex.

CEMENTOMA

True cementoma is a mass of cementum and resembles dentinoma radiologically.

PERIAPICAL CEMENTIFYING DYSPLASIA (PCD)

The so called CEMENTOMA is to be considered as a fibroosseous lesion (described under the heading of periapical lesions).

BENIGN CEMENTOBLASTOMA

1. It occurs in younger patients of about 25 years of age.
2. This lesion is seen more frequently in the mandibular second premolar and first molar region.
3. Females are more commonly affected than males.
4. It is derived from cementoblasts in the periodontal ligament space and gives rise to a bulbous deposition of cementum surrounding the teeth.
5. Patient's complaint of pain may be due to periodontal infection around the root of the affected tooth and the lesion, and is unlikely to respond to endodontic treatment.

Radiographic Features

(i) Cementoblastoma appears as dense radiopaque mass covering lower half of the roots, through which the roots cannot be traced (Fig.10.3).

(ii) Surrounding this radiopaque mass, a radiolucent halo is visible.

(iii) The teeth in question are vital and the patient may get a painful swelling.

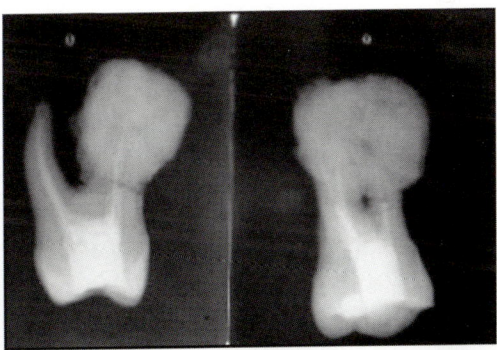

Fig. 10.3: A Cementoblastoma attached to the root of the molar.

D/D:

(a) Periapical cemental dysplasia: It has a predilection for lower anterior region in women aged more than 40 years. The lesion passes through three stages, namely the early radiolucent, intermediate mixed and the late radiopaque stage.

(b) Hypercementosis: It is the bulbous enlargement of the root around the apex in a uniform manner from the CE junction.

(c) Other conditions such as condensing osteitis, enostosis and torus must be differentiated from cementoblastoma.

COMPLEX COMPOSITE ODONTOME

1. As the name suggests it is a composite lesion consisting of enamel, dentine and cementum. There is no morphodifferentiation and the lesion appears as a single complex mass with haphazard distribution of enamel, dentine and cementum.

2. Seen in the upper anterior and in the lower first molar regions.

3. It may be associated with unerupted/impacted tooth.

4. The impacted tooth may be malformed, dilacerated or pushed close to the lower border.

Radiographic Appearance

(i) Complex composite odontome appears as a dense radiopaque mass the density of which is equal to that of the dental tissues (Fig. 10.4).

(ii) It is surrounded by a radiolucent halo suggestive of a fibrous capsule. This radiolucent halo is in turn surrounded by corticated bone.

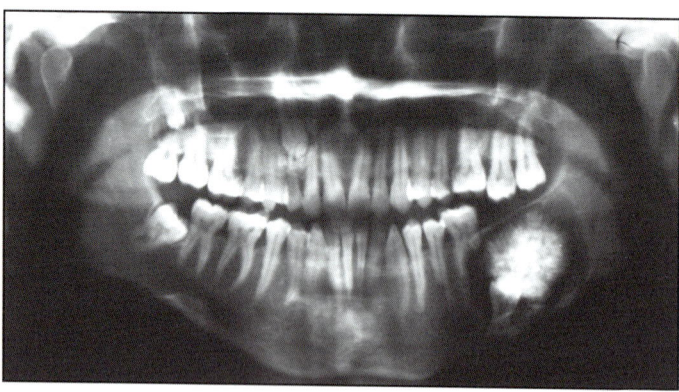

Fig. 10.4: OPG showing a large complex composite odontome in the mandible. Also note the presence of an impacted maxillary right canine with compound odontome.

Complication of odontomas: It can result in fracture of mandible during its removal.

D/D: Osteoma (Osteoma is composed of bone and attached to the bone with no fibrous capsule).

COMPOUND COMPOSITE ODONTOME

1. This is also a composite lesion made up of two or more tooth like bodies with enamel-capped crowns known as ***denticles.***

2. They are seen in the region of upper and lower canines and first premolars.

3. The lesion may be associated with impacted teeth. In such cases it is usually seen coronal to the impacted teeth.

4. Each denticle is surrounded by a fibrous capsule and the entire odontome is in turn surrounded by a fibrous capsule. Thus, it is possible to separate out a number of teeth like bodies with enamel and dentine during the surgery.

Radiographic Features

This condition presents as multiple radiopaque bodies surrounded by a radiolucent fibrous capsule which is in turn surrounded by a corticated border (Figs 10.4 and 10.5).

Complication: One or two denticles may be left behind.

Cystic varieties of both, complex as well as compound odontomes exist. They appear on the radiograph as large radiolucent lesions around the radiopaque masses.

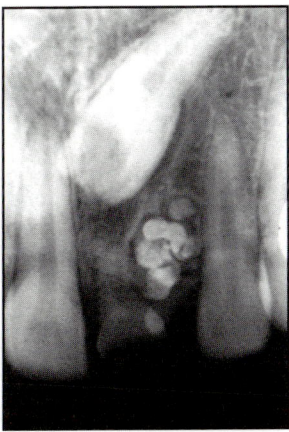

Fig. 10.5: Radiograph showing a compound composite odontome.

GEMINATED ODONTOME

1. Gemination is due to the division of one tooth bud.
2. It may manifest as a single large tooth with a notch in the incisal edge. Sometimes the notch becomes deeper so that even the pulp chamber appears notched.
3. Occasionally two separate crowns with a single root may be seen on the radiograph.

DILATED ODONTOME

DENS IN DENTE (DENS INVAGINATUS)

1. Etiology: Dens in dente are formed due to invagination of the outer enamel layer into the developing tooth material.
2. The most commonly affected teeth are the maxillary lateral incisors.
3. The crown appears peg-shaped with an aperture on the incisal edge.
4. This tooth invariably has a periapical lesion because it has an enamel lined tract within the tooth connected to the aperture in the crown which provides free access to micro organisms and food debris.

Radiographic Features

i. Radiograph shows *tooth within a tooth* appearance because of enamel lined tract within the tooth (Fig 10.6).

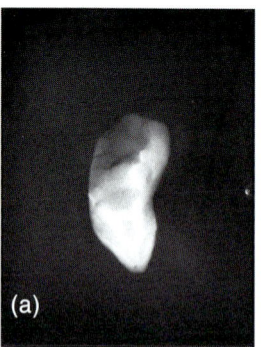 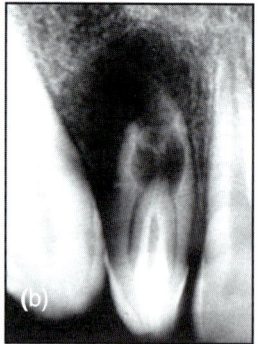

Figs 10.6a and b: (a) Radiograph showing a dilated odontome in the lateral incisor. (b) Radiograph of dens in dente resembling Fleur-de-lys.

ii. It is also called as Invaginated odontome.

iii. H.M.Worth has described two more types of dilated odontome.

– A root dilation resembling an inverted open umbrella.

– Fleur-de-lys which resembles the French emblem (Fig. 10.6a).

NEOPLASIA

According to Rupert Willis, neoplasm is *"An abnormal mass of tissue, the growth of which exceeds and is uncoordinated with that of the normal tissues and persists in the same excessive manner after cessation of the stimuli that evoked the change."*

Neoplasms may be classified as benign and malignant. The benign tumors are usually slow growing and do not have a fatal outcome, whereas malignant tumors are aggressive, spread to distant sites and often have a fatal outcome.

Difference between Benign and Malignant Tumors

BENIGN TUMORS	MALIGNANT TUMORS
I. MACROSCOPIC	
They are usually single and loculated.	They are multiple and diffuse
Lesions are round, elliptical, pedunculated or sessile	Lesions have an irregular shape
Benign tumors are encapsulated	Malignant tumors are not encapsulated
They exhibit a slow growth	They exhibit a rapid growth
Necrosis is uncommon	Necrosis is common
Their removal is easy	Their removal is difficult
Lymph node involvement is not seen	Lymph nodes are involved, hard and fixed
They cause root resorption and displacement of teeth	This is rare with malignant tumors.
Metastasis is absent	Metastasis may occur to distant sites
Recurrence is uncommon	Recurrence is common
Benign tumors usually do not have a fatal outcome	Malignant tumors usually have a fatal outcome

Contd.

Contd.

BENIGN TUMORS	MALIGNANT TUMORS
They have a smooth surface with normal mucosa	They have a surface which is irregular and thrown into exophytic growth/ulcerative lesions.
Fetid odor is absent	Fetid odour present
II. MICROSCOPIC	
Tumor cells are similar to parent cells	Tumor cells are undifferentiated/anaplastic
Tumor is confined by a fibrous capsule	There is no well-defined capsule that confines the tumor
Tumor cells do not penetrate the connective tissue	Tumor cells penetrate the connective tissue
Nuclei appear normal and do not show dysplastic changes	Abnormal nuclei are seen with dysplastic changes such as abnormal mitosis, increased nucleus/cytoplasmic ratio.
III. RADIOGRAPHIC	
Benign tumors show expansion Margins are well defined	Malignant tumors show destruction Margins are ill-defined and irregular (bays and promontories)
They cause root resorption which appears smooth and blunt	They cause irregular spiked resorption of the roots
Benign tumors displace the anatomical landmarks, e.g. inferior dental canal, maxillary sinus	Malignant tumors destroy the anatomical landmarks, e.g. break in the floor of antrum.
Pathological fractures are rare	Large lesions frequently cause pathological fractures

The benign tumors include:
1. Ameloblastoma
2. Giant cell lesions:
   – Benign giant cell granuloma
   – Reparative giant cell
   – Giant cell tumor of bone
   – Giant cell tumor of bone associated with hyperparathyroidism
     Giant cell epulis
3. AOT
4. CEOT

5. Papilloma
6. Fibroma
   – in soft tissue
   – in bone: central, odontogenic, ossifying
7. Epulis
   – fibroid
   – giant cell-vascular
8. Hemangioma
   – Sturge-Weber syndrome
   – Osler-Rendu-Weber syndrome
9. Odontogenic myxoma
10. Lipoma
11. Chondroma
12. Osteoma
    – compact/ivory osteoma
    – cancellous osteoma
    – osteoid osteoma
13. Hyperostosis/exostosis
    – torus palatinus
    – torus mandibularis
14. Enostoses/ bone whorl.

ODONTOGENIC TUMORS

WHO classification of odontogenic tumors.

A. Benign Tumors

I. Odontogenic epithelial tumors without ectomesenchymal induction:
   (a) Ameloblastoma.
   (b) Squamous odontogenic tumor.
   (c) Calcifying epithelial odontogenic tumor (CEOT)/Pindborg tumor.
   (d) Adenomatoid odontogenic tumor (AOT).
II. Odontogenic epithelial tumors with ectomesenchymal induction with or without hard tissue formation:
   (a) Ameloblastic fibroma.

    (b) Ameloblastic fibro-odontoma

    (c) Odontoameloblastoma

    (d) CEOC

    (e) Compound odontome

    (f) Complex odontome

  III. Odontogenic ectomesenchymal tumors with or without induction of odontogenic epithelium:

    (a) Odontogenic fibroma

    (b) Odontogenic myxoma

    (c) Cementoblastoma

B. Malignant Tumors

  I. Odontogenic carcinomas

    (a) Malignant ameloblastoma

    (b) Primary intraalveolar carcinoma

    (c) Clear cell odontogenic tumor

    (d) Ghost cell odontogenic carcinoma

  II. Odontogenic sarcomas

    (a) Ameloblastic fibrosarcoma

    (b) Ameloblastic fibro-dentino-sarcoma

    (c) Ameloblastic odonto-sarcoma

AMELOBLASTOMA

According to Robinson, ameloblastoma is defined as 'a tumor of the odontogenic epithelium, which is unicentric, non-functional, intermittent in growth, anatomically benign and clinically persistent lesion which does not undergo differentiation to the extent of hard tissue formation'.

Origin:

  (i) Ameloblastoma arises from the enamel organ or the basal cell layer of epithelium.

 (ii) Some lesions such as the mural ameloblastoma may arise from the lining of the dentigerous cyst.

(iii) Certain lesions originate from the basal cells of the epithelium of the jaw.

Types of Ameloblastomas

Depending on the location, ameloblastomas may be of the following types:

    I – Peripheral (extraosseous)

    II – Intraosseous

    III – Pituitary ameloblastoma arising from heterotropic epithelium in the Rathke's pouch

Depending on their structure, they may be:

    I – Solid or

    II – Cystic

According to the histological pattern, they can be classified as:

    I – Follicular

    II – Plexiform

    III – Desmoplastic

    IV – Acanthomatous

    V – Granular cell

    VI – Basal.

Malignant ameloblastoma: It is defined as that particular ameloblastoma which has given evidence of truly malignant behaviour judged chiefly by the occurrence of metastasis, but in which the metastatic lesions have no significant differences from the primary tumor. In other words, the metastatic tumor still resembles the primary tumor and has no histological evidence of malignant transformation.

Ameloblastic carcinoma: It is defined as that type of ameloblastoma in which there has been obvious histologically malignant transformation of the epithelial component and in which the tumor has behaved in a malignant fashion, so that the metastatic lesions do not resemble the primary odontogenic tumor, but rather to a less differentiated carcinoma, usually an epidermoid carcinoma.

Mural ameloblastoma: It is a unicystic variant arising from the lining of dentigerous cyst. It is further classified into:

Type I   – Lesion with simple epithelial lining resembling ameloblastoma.

Type II   – Lesions with a mass of ameloblastoma proliferating into the lumen of the cyst.

Type III   – Invasive tumor growing into the connective tissue wall.

Clinical Features

1. Age: Ameloblastomas are usually seen in adults over 30 years of age.
2. Sex: Males are more commonly affected than females.
3. The mandible is more commonly affected than the maxilla. In the mandible, the molar and ramus areas have a high predilection. When ameloblastoma affects the maxilla, it is usually very aggressive and leads to serious complications due to involvement of the nasopharynx, maxillary sinus, orbit and the base of skull.
4. They present as slow growing asymptomatic swelling which may give rise to severe deformity.
5. The mucous membrane over the swelling is normal unless traumatized by opposing teeth.
6. It gives rise to expansion of buccal and lingual cortical plates.

Radiographic Features

As described by H.M.Worth, 4 types of appearances are seen. These appearances have been diagrammatically represented in Fig. 10.7a.

1. **Unicystic type:** It appears as a unilocular radiolucency resembling a cyst. However unlike a cyst, it causes a break or discontinuity in the peripheral cortex and may even show trabeculae within the lumen.
2. **Spider variety:** This is the most common appearance where the lesion is seen as a large radiolucent area with scalloped borders. From the centre of the lumen, coarse strands of trabeculae radiate peripherally giving size to a *gross caricature of a spider* (Fig. 10.9).
3. **Multilocular radiolucency:** Ameloblastomas may be seen as multilocular radiolucencies having a *soap-bubble appearance* or *bunch of grapes* type of appearance (Fig. 10.7b).
4. **Solid ameloblastoma:** It is one which has not undergone cystic degeneration. Hence multiple small radiolucencies are seen surrounded by hexagonal or polygonal thick walled bony cortices giving rise to a *honeycomb* appearance (Fig. 10.8).
5. If it occurs in the mandible it may spread to the inferior border giving rise to fracture. They also have a high rate of recurrence.

Treatment: Extensive surgical treatment is required. Radiotherapy is contraindicated because it may result in malignant transformation of the lesion.

Differential Diagnosis: Cyst and tumor radiographically.

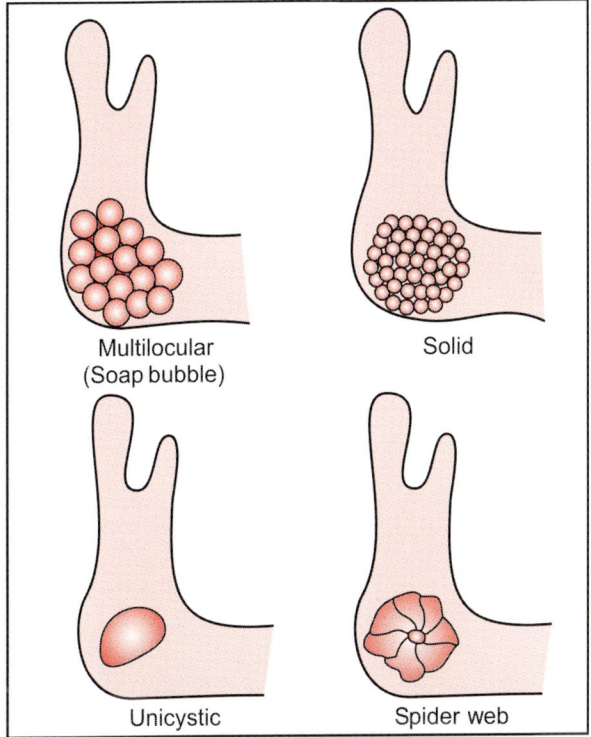

Fig. 10.7a: Different radiographic appearances of ameloblastoma.

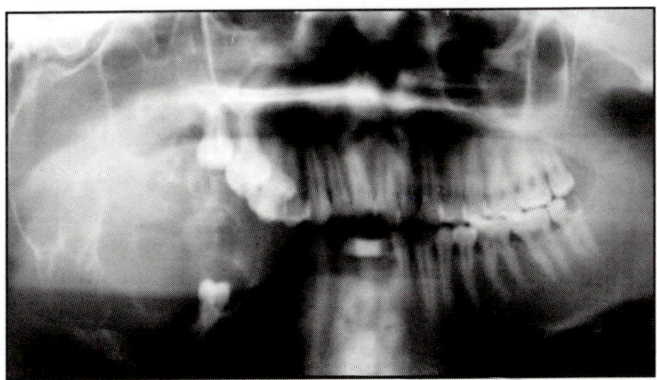

Fig. 10.7b: OPG showing an ameloblastoma appearing as multilocular soap-bubble appearance.

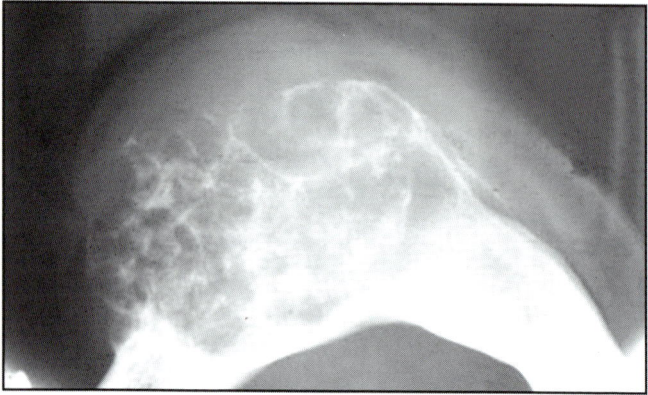

Fig. 10.8: Occlusal view showing an ameloblastoma appearing as multilocular honeycomb appearance.

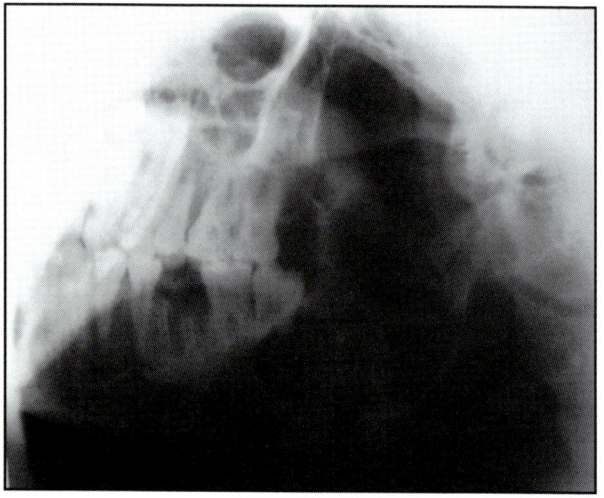

Fig. 10.9: Ameloblastoma appearing as a gross caricature of a spider.

The differentiating points between a cyst and benign tumor are as follows.

CYST	BENIGN TUMOR
The radiolucency of a cyst is more due to its fluid content.	The radiolucency of a tumor is less due to its tissue content.
The borders are smooth, round, continuous and corticated.	The borders of the lesion are scalloped.

Contd.

Contd.

Trabeculae are usually absent within the lesion.	Trabeculae may be present within the lesion.
Septae are absent.	Septae are present.
Cysts cause only buccal expansion except in primordial cyst which may cause lingual expansion.	Tumors cause buccal and lingual expansion.
Root resorption and displacement are less common.	Root resorption and displacement are more marked.
Egg shell crackling may be present with large cyst.	No egg shell crackling is noted.

BENIGN GIANT CELL GRANULOMA

(Previously known as reparative giant cell granuloma)

Origin: The tumor originates from osteoblasts/odontoblasts, i.e. giant cells.

Clinical Features

1. Age: Giant cell granuloma usually occurs in the younger age group with an average age of 15–16 yrs.
2. Sex: Females are more frequently affected than males.
   Site: The region anterior to the first molar is the preferred site. This may be because; odontoblasts which have caused resorption of deciduous teeth are present at this site from which the tumor arises.
3. The tumor exhibits a rapid growth and appears as a fleshy swelling
4. Lesion is painless, but it may bleed spontaneously.
5. Mobility and displacement of teeth may be present.

Radiographic Findings

(i) Giant cell granuloma appears as a radiolucent lesion in the anterior portion of the jaw, often crossing the midline (Figs 10.10 and 10.11). The margins of the lesion may be regular, irregular or corticated.

(ii) The lumen shows the presence of thin, delicate trabeculae described as wispy striae.

(iii) Root resorption and expansion of the cortical plates are also common findings.

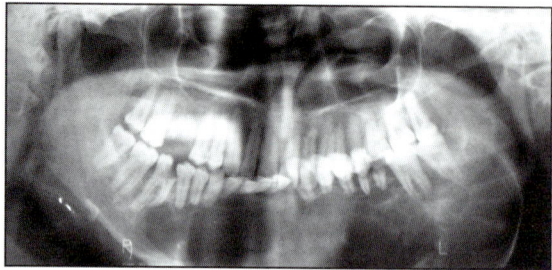

Fig. 10.10: OPG showing a large giant cell granuloma in the mandible.

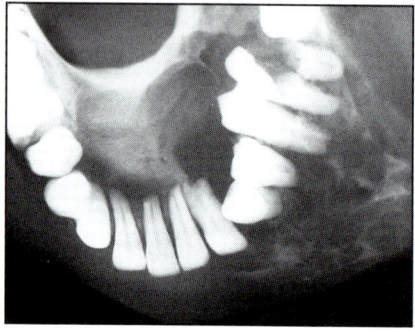

Fig. 10.11: Occlusal radiograph of the same case in Fig. 10.10 showing marked expansion of cortices and displacement of teeth.

GIANT CELL TUMOR WITH HYPERPARATHYROIDISM (Brown Tumor)

Giant cell tumors are associated with hyperparathyroidism and occur in young females. The lesion presents as a large osteolytic lesion in the jaws. Generalized disappearance of lamina dura may be another finding in such cases.

Due to increase in the levels of parathyroid hormone, calcium is withdrawn from the bone. Serum calcium and alkaline phosphatase levels are raised.

They are also called as brown tumor, because the lesion in a cut section appears brown due to areas of hemorrhage. These tumors heal when the underlying pathology is corrected.

GIANT CELL EPULIS

They appear as pedunculated reddish swellings which bleed easily and do not show calcification on the radiograph as opposed to fibroid epulis.

ADENOMATOID ODONTOGENIC TUMOR (AOT)/ADENO AMELOBLASTOMA

It is a benign odontogenic epithelial tumor arising from the enamel organ epithelium.

Types of AOT

Based upon their location in the jaws, they may be:

I – Central or

II – Peripheral

The central tumors may be further divided into:

(a) Follicular type which are associated with impacted teeth, and

(b) Extrafollicular type which are not associated with impacted teeth.

Clinical Features

1. AOT has a special predilection for the maxillary anterior region of the jaw in young females.
2. Lesions present as slow growing, gradually enlarging painless mass.
3. Often a tooth may be missing in the region affected by the tumor.

Radiographic Features

(i) A common presentation of AOT is pericoronal radiolucency with well-defined margins.

(ii) The interior of the lesion may contain many small radiopaque flecks giving rise to *Milky Way lumen appearance* to the lesion (Fig. 10.12).

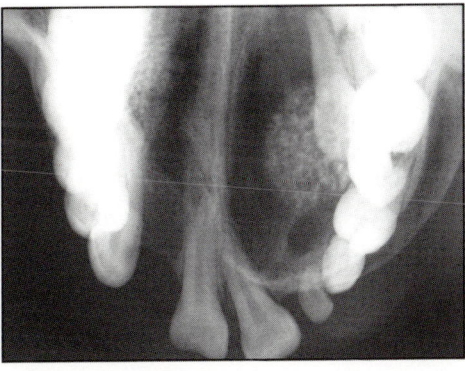

Fig. 10.12: Radiograph showing an impacted tooth with pericoronal radiolucency and radiopaque flecks within the lesion.

(iii) The enlarging tumor can cause expansion of the cortices and displacement of teeth, while root resorption is rare.

Differential Diagnosis: Dentigerous cyst (The radiolucency is attached to the cervical region of the tooth and covers only the crown of the tooth), CEOT, odontomes, etc.

PINDBORG'S TUMOR/CALCIFYING EPITHELIAL ODONTOGENIC TUMOR (CEOT)

1. These are rare tumors that occur in the jaws and produce mineralized substances within their lumen.
2. They may be located within the bone or may also have an extraosseous form.
3. Slow growing expansion of the jaws resulting in a hard palpable swelling in the premolar-molar region is a presenting feature.
4. The radiographic appearance is of a unilocular or multilocular lesion with internal radiopaque areas having a *driven snow* appearance.
5. **Differential diagnosis:** AOT, ameloblastic fibrodontome, CEOC.

ODONTOGENIC MYXOMA

1. Myxomas are rare benign tumors occurring only in the facial bones. The tumors arise from the odontogenic ectomesenchyme and resemble dental papilla histologically.
2. The lesions are not encapsulated and have a jelly-like consistency. They tend to infiltrate into the surrounding tissues, thereby resulting in high recurrence rate of the tumor.
3. Myxomas affect the mandible more often than the maxilla and present as slow growing painless swelling.
4. Radiologically, they are seen as well-defined multilocular lesions, sometimes associated with an impacted tooth. The internal structure is made up of thin, straight bony trabeculae arranged at right angles to the periphery giving rise to a *strings of a tennis racket* like appearance (Fig. 10.13).

OSTEOMA

Osteomas are benign tumors arising from membranous bones of the face and skull. They originate from the periosteum of the bone and grow outwards or inward into the sinuses.

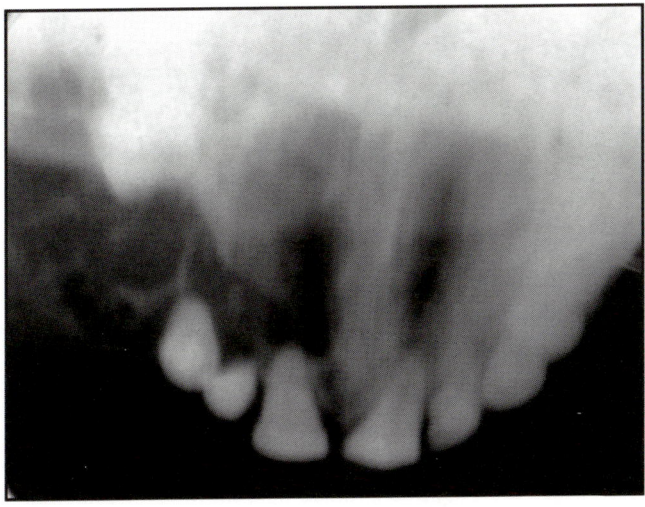

Fig. 10.13: Occlusal view of a myxoma in the maxilla.

Types of Osteoma

Based on their structure, osteomas are of three types:

   (i) Ivory osteoma, composed of compact bone.

  (ii) Cancellous osteoma composed of cancellous bone.

 (iii) Osteoid osteoma.

1. Osteomas present as hard painless swellings in the jaws bones which are attached to the jaw bone by means of a pedicle or a wide base.

2. The lower border of the mandible in the posterior jaw and the lingual cortical plate are the most common sites for development of osteomas.

3. Radiographically, they appear as dense radiopaque structures (Fig.10.14). Cancellous osteomas may show the presence of internal trabeculae.

Gardner's syndrome: This is a hereditary syndrome caused due to mutation of the APC (Adenoid Polyposis Coli) gene, characterized by multiple osteomas, cutaneous sebaceous cysts, subcutaneous fibromas and multiple intestinal polyps. These polyps have a high tendency to undergo malignant transformation. Another important feature of this syndrome is the presence of multiple impacted supernumerary teeth in the jaws.

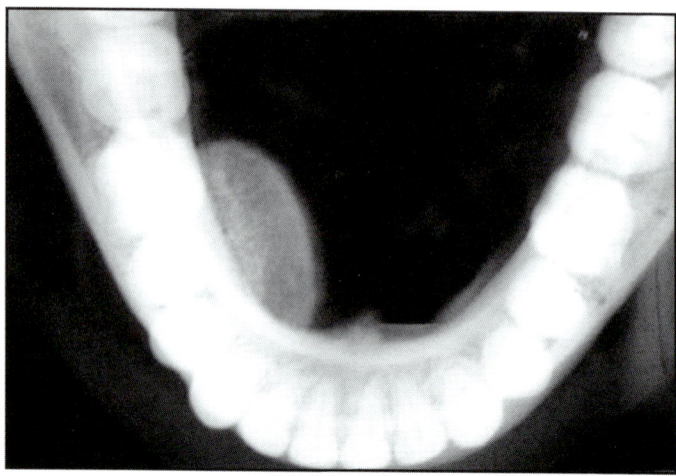

Fig. 10.14: Occlusal radiograph showing an osteoma.

HEMANGIOMA

Hemangioma is a benign tumor originating from the blood vessels. Some investigators believe this to be a hamartoma since it has a limited capacity for growth and stops growing after certain periods.

Clinical Features

1. Hemangiomas may occur exclusively in the soft tissues or within the bone.
2. Lesions are often present at the time of birth and grow until puberty.
3. The lesions involving the soft tissues appear as bluish red, soft fluctuant swellings (Fig. 10.15). They may exhibit blanching on palpation (diascopy).
4. The swelling may be pulsatile and bruit can be heard if auscultated.
5. If traumatized, hemangiomas bleed extensively and the bleeding is difficult to control.
6. Lesions present within the bone cause expansion of the bone.
7. When the tooth in the region is pressed, it sinks below the occlusal level within the socket and rebounds after some time. This is called a *pumping tooth.*
8. Intra bony hemangiomas can present with abnormal oozing of blood from the gingival crevice even in the absence of any local factors.

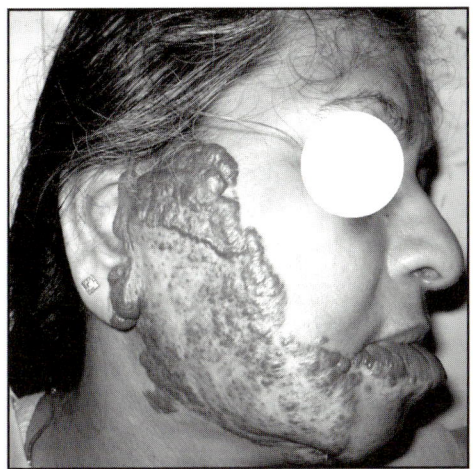

Fig. 10.15: Clinical appearance of hemangioma.

Radiographic Appearance

(i) Hemangiomas may be seen as a unilocular or multilocular radiolucency.

(ii) The characteristic picture is the *spokes of wheel* appearance with radial arrangement of trabeculae.

(iii) Sometimes, radiopaque bodies may be seen within the lesion which represent the calcified thrombi called *phleboliths* (Fig. 10.16).

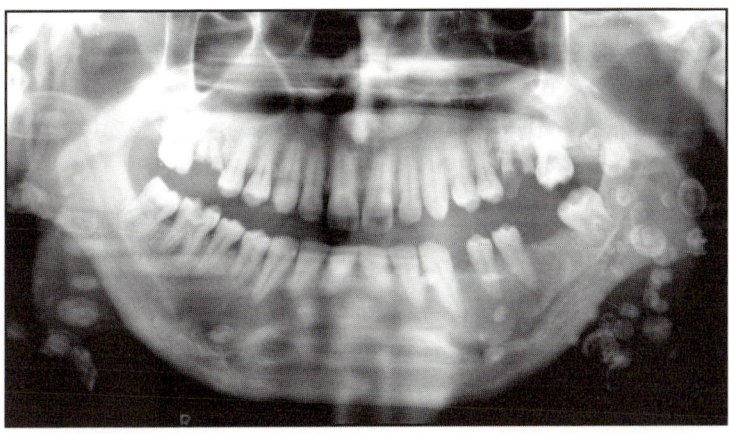

Fig. 10.16: Radiograph showing phleboliths of a hemangioma (in another patient).

(iv) When hemangiomas occur within the mandibular canal, they cause the canal to enlarge in a serpiginous fashion. The mandibular and mental foramen may be enlarged.

(v) The lesion can cause root resorption and displacement. Also the teeth in the vicinity of a hemangioma may appear to be larger in size, show signs of root development and eruption earlier than other teeth.

Treatment

Hemangiomas can be treated by injection of sclerosing agents such as sodium tetradecyl sulphate into the lesion. Cryosurgery and surgery with ligation of the external carotid artery can also be done to treat the lesions.

Sturge-Weber Syndrome (encephalo-trigeminal angiomatosis)

This syndrome is an unusual congenital disease characterized by the combination of venous hemangioma of the leptomeninges over the cerebral cortex with ipsilateral angiomatous lesions over the face and sometimes the skull, jaws and oral soft tissues. Intracranial calcification and convulsive disorders are also features of this syndrome. These patients may also have gingival enlargement secondary to anticonvulsive drug therapy.

SUGGESTED READING AND REFERENCES

1. Oral Radiology—Principles and Interpretation: White and Pharoah, 5th edition.
2. Essentials of Dental Radiography and Radiology—Eric Whaites, 3rd edition.
3. Principles and Practice of Oral Radiographic Interpretations—H.M. Worth.
4. Differential Diagnosis of Oral Lesions—Wood and Goaz.
5. Panoramic Radiology—Langland.

CHAPTER 11

Malignant Tumors

Malignant tumors unlike the benign tumors are very aggressive in nature and often have a fatal outcome. Harrison has defined malignant tumor by a few characteristics which describe how cancer cells act differently from their normal counterparts.

1. **Clonality:** Malignant tumor originates from genetic changes in a single cell which proliferates to form a clone of malignant cells.
2. **Autonomy:** Growth is autonomous and not regulated by normal biochemical and physical influences in the environment.
3. **Anaplasia:** There is lack of normal, coordinated cell differentiation.
4. **Metastasis:** Malignant tumor develops the capacity for discontinuous growth and dissemination to different parts of the body.

Primary malignant tumor: These are tumors that arise de novo.

Secondary/metastatic malignant tumors: These are tumors that develop at a distant site due to spread of primary tumor.

Carcinogenesis is believed to be due to two factors: *Initiation* and *promotion*.

Initiation factors give rise to somatic changes in the cell, thus making it more prone or vulnerable to the promoting factors, e.g. application of urethane on mice does not result in cancers but urethane application followed by croton oil application show malignant changes.

The malignant cells display what is called as lack of contact inhibition with results in continuous proliferation. Some authors also describe cancer as growth of new cells which proliferate without control and serve no useful function.

The main carcinogenic agents include:

1. *Chemical agents:* Carcinoma of scrotum found in chimney sweepers.

   Exposure to aniline dye can cause carcinoma of the bladder Butyl yellow, Polycyclic aromatic hydrocarbon, Tar, etc. are also some chemical that are known to cause cancers.

2. *Viruses:* Bittner's milk factor is a viral carcinogen known to cause transfer of cancers via mother's milk in mice.

   Epstein-Barr virus (EBV) causes Burkitt's lymphoma in African children.

3. *Ionizing radiation,* e.g. X-rays: Carcinoma of lung common in miners working in cobalt mines.

   Malignancy commonly seen in people painting fluorescent watch dials.

   Leukemia is common in survivors of atomic explosions and radiologists, e.g. Dr. Edmund Kells an early radiologist suffered from cancer of the skin due to exposure to radiation.

4. *Hormonal factors:* Carcinoma of breast, cervix, prostrate is associated with abnormal hormonal changes.

Modes of Spread of Malignancies

1. Infiltration: Malignant tumors are not capsulated and the cells infiltrate into the surrounding tissues. While benign tumors have a well-defined capsule and do not spread into the adjacent tissue.

2. Lymphatic spread:
   (a) Local lymphatic permeation (along vessel wall).
   (b) Lymphatic embolism (tumor cells forming the embolus).
       Most carcinomas spread by lymphatics.

3. Blood borne spread: Malignant cells may enter the vascular channels and spread to distant sites. Most sarcomas spread by this route.

4. Spread through natural spaces, e.g. renal pelvis to bladder.

5. Through the serous body cavities

6. Inoculation: The surgeon might accidentally implant malignant cells at the site from which skin graft is taken.

7. Perineural spread, e.g. adenoid cystic carcinomas of the minor salivary gland.
8. Perivascular spread.

DIAGNOSTIC AIDS

1. Clinical examination:
   (a) Chronic ulcer with everted margins
   (b) Fixed ulcer
   (c) Exophytic growth
   (d) Erythroplakia or speckled leukoplakias which are pre malignant lesions with reddish granular area.
   (e) Fixed lymph node.
2. Chemiluminescence—Vizilite and velscope.
3. X-rays, tomography, ultrasound, full body scanning.
4. Biopsy
5. Cytologic smear, brush biopsy
6. FNAC – Fine Needle Aspiration Cytology
7. FNAB – Fine Needle Aspiration Biopsy
8. Use of toluidine blue.

Grading of Malignant Tumors

Cancers may be graded microscopically or macroscopically. Macroscopically the tumor can be graded as being exophytic, fungative, ulcerative, invasive, etc. while the former two types are believed to be less aggressive and have a better prognosis; the latter two appearances are usually suggestive of a grave prognosis. However a more reliable method of grading tumors is on the basis of the degree of anaplasia as detected microscopically. The tumor may be graded as follows:

Grade I   :   Well-differentiated tumors (25% anaplastic cells).
Grade II   :   Moderately differentiated tumors (25–50% anaplastic cells).
Grade III :   Moderately differentiated tumors (50–75% anaplastic cells).
Grade IV   :   Poorly differentiated (more than 75% anaplastic cells).

Staging of Tumors

Staging of tumors determines the extent of spread of tumor in the body. Staging can be predominantly assessed by clinical examination. However the role of diagnostic imaging and pathologic examination is also valuable in the staging and malignant diseases.

TNM staging

The tumor, node, metastasis (TNM) staging was proposed by the American Joint Committee on Cancer (AJCC).

T is determined by the size of the tumor.

N indicates the presence of lymph node metastasis.

M indicates the presence of distant metastasis.

This staging system has combined T, N and M to stage the lesions as 1 to 4.

The **TNM staging** for the **tumors** of the **oral cavity** is as follows:

T   :   Size of the tumor

T_{1S} :   CA in situ

T_2 :   Tumor size <2 cm

T_3 :   Tumor size >2 cm, but <4 cm

T_4 :   Tumor size >4 cm with invasion into the adjacent tissues

N   :   Cervical lymph node metastasis

N_0 :   No nodal involvement is detected

N_1 :   Single ipsilateral node < 3 cm

N_{2a} :   Single ipsilateral node < 6 cm

N_{2b} :   Multiple ipsilateral nodes > 3 cm, but < 6 cm

N_{2c} :   Bilateral/contralateral nodes < 6 cm

N_{3a} :   Ipsilateral nodes > 6 cm

N_{3b} :   Bilateral nodes > 6 cm

M   :   Metastasis

M_0 :   Unknown metastasis

M_1 :   Metastasis present

Staging

Stage 1 : $T_1N_0M_0$

Stage 2 : $T_2N_0M_0$

Stage 3 : $T_3N_0M_0$

$T_1/T_2/T_3,N_1M_0$

Stage 4 : T_4, any N,M_0

any $T,N_2/N_3,M_0$

any T or N,M_1

Further in order to simplify and make the staging more specific for a particular region, the AJCC has recommended an individualized staging system for cancers in the various areas of the oral cavity and the head and neck region.

SQUAMOUS CELL CARCINOMA

Squamous cell carcinomas are the most common malignant tumors occurring in the oral cavity. In most cases, they arise from a pre-existing premalignant lesion such as leukoplakia, erythroplakia or OSMF.

Clinical Features

1. Squamous cell carcinoma appears as an ulcerative lesion of long-standing duration with everted margins.
2. The ulcer is fixed to the underlying tissues. Fixity is due to infiltration of the tumor tissue into the underlying connective tissue.
3. Carcinoma may also manifest as an exophytic growth with rough, pebbled, irregular surface described as a cauliflower like growth.
4. Cervical lymph nodes may be hard, palpable and fixed.
5. Pain is not a common feature, but the function of the affected part is restricted, e.g. tongue movements and speech are affected in carcinoma of tongue.

Radiographic Findings

(i) Squamous cell carcinoma is a lesion which starts in the soft tissues lining the vestibule or other parts of the oral cavity. It is not a primary lesion of the bone, but a lesion which secondarily affects the bone. Hence, in the early stages, when not more than 30% calcium is removed from the bone, changes are not apparent radiographically. (A radionuclide scan may help in the diagnosis during this stage of the disease.)

(ii) As malignancy progresses, it erodes or removes the superficial part of the bone giving rise to an osteolytic defect. This defect may be small or large, superficial or deep.

(iii) This osteolytic defect appears on the radiograph as an area of radiolucency with ragged and ill-defined permeative borders. Such an appearance is described as *bays and promontories like appearance* (Fig. 11.1).

(iv) The most characteristic feature of malignant tumor is the lack of corticated margins.

(v) Extensive destruction of bone may give rise to pathological fracture of the jaw.

(vi) The teeth in the area of involvement are devoid of bone support and appear as *floating or hanging* teeth (Fig. 11.1).

(vii) Sometimes there may be root resorption which appears irregular and spiked unlike the smooth resorption seen with benign tumors.

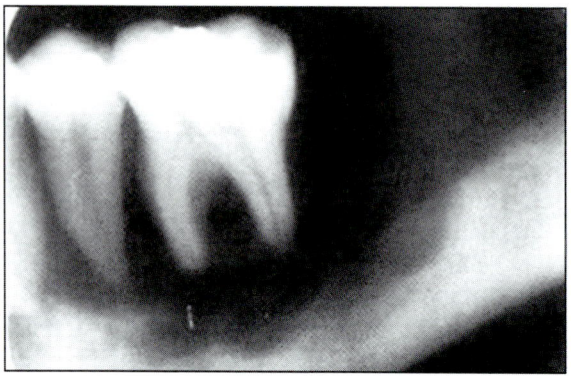

Fig. 11.1: Radiograph showing floating tooth and bays and promontories like appearance caused due to squamous cell carcinoma.

D.D.

(a) *Periodontal disease:* Bone loss associated with periodontal disease is usually parallel to the original lamina dura and the radiographs show areas of sclerosis adjacent to the osteolytic lesion suggestive of infection. But a malignant tumor has an irregular margin without sclerosis.

(b) *Osteomyelitis:* Periosteal reaction and sequestrum formation are usually present in osteomyelitis, but absent in a malignant tumor.

D.D. for '*floating tooth appearance*' include Squamous cell carcinoma, eosinophilic granuloma, early stages of cherubism, osteomyelitis, severe periodontitis.

METASTATIC CARCINOMA

1. They are the most common tumors affecting the bones, but relatively rare in the jaws.

2. The most common bones to be affected by metastasis are the skull bones and the vertebra. When the jaws are affected, the main route of spread to the jaws is through the *pre vertebral veins of Batson*.

3. In the jaws, mandible is a more common site for metastatic tumors. The common source of primary tumors that spread to the jaws are breast, lung, kidney, thyroid, prostate, colon and stomach.

4. Metastatic tumors may be painless. Occasionally, the patient may give an unsolicited complaint of numbness or paresthesia without any apparent cause.

5. Radiographically, metastatic malignancies can be of three types: osteolytic, osteoblastic, osteosclerotic. Tumors of prostate and breast are osteoblastic and appear radiopaque due to multiple radiopaque foci, more so if the tumor responds to hormone therapy.

The various radiographic appearances of metastatic malignancies are (Fig 11.2):

(i) Solitary well-defined radiolucency.
(ii) Solitary poorly defined radiolucency.
(iii) Multiple separate poorly defined radiolucency.
(iv) Multiple punched out radiolucency.
(v) Radiopaque masses due to sclerosis or bone formation.
(vi) Salt and pepper appearance in widely disseminated bone lesions.
(vii) Dense radiopaque solitary mass.

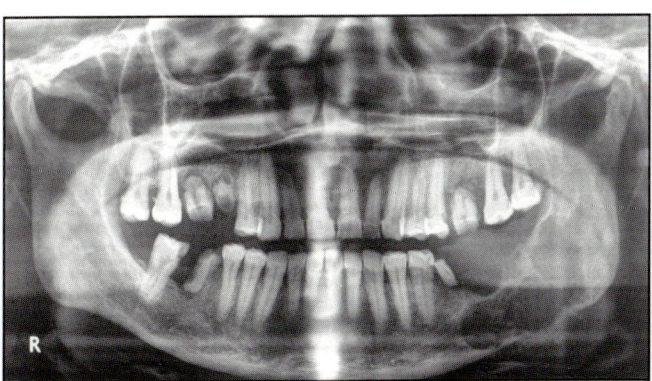

Fig. 11.2: OPG showing metastatic thyroid carcinoma in the left mandible.

Radionuclide scans including Positron Emission Tomography (PET) play an important role in the detection of metastatic tumors.

OSTEOSARCOMA

1. Osteosarcoma is a malignant tumor of the bone. It presents as rapidly growing swelling of the jaws and may be accompanied by pain, tenderness, erythema and ulceration of the mucosa.
2. The posterior part of the mandible is more commonly affected than the maxilla.
3. It appears as ill-defined radiolucent lesion without any evidence of sclerosis. The internal structure may appear as mixed radiolucent and radiopaque or completely radiopaque.
4. Periosteal reaction in the form of *hair on end*, *sunray spicules* or *Codman's triangle* may be present which are highly suggestive of osteosarcoma (Fig. 11.3). Osteogenic sarcoma is basically a bone forming tumor involving the osteoblasts and therefore the osteoblasts present sub periosteally tend to lay down the bone in different patterns as described by H.M. Worth. The most common periosteal reaction of these, is the sunray appearance. The

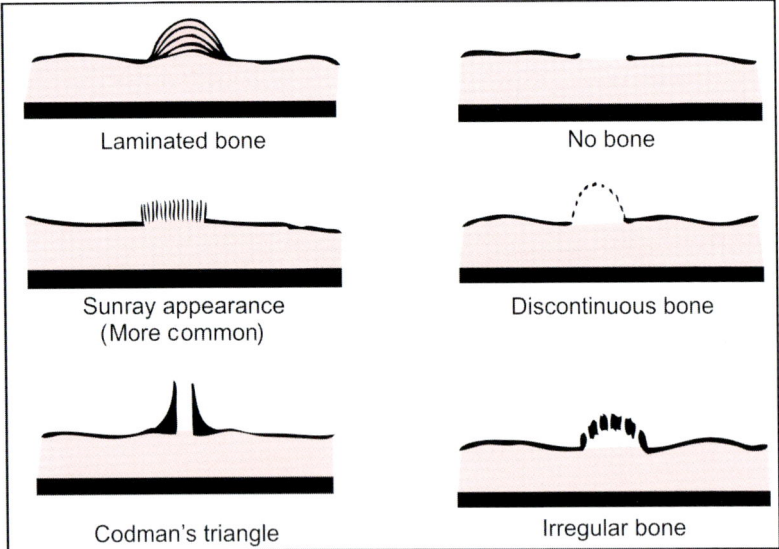

Fig. 11.3: Various types of periosteal reactions that may occur in osteosarcoma.

Codman's triangle is a triangular shape of bone deposited in the space between the original cortex of the bone, elevated periosteum and the tumor mass.

5. The cortices of the mandibular canal and the lamina dura of the teeth may be destroyed by the lesion.

6. The periodontal ligament space of the teeth in the affected portion of the jaw appears to be widened. This is called as *Garrington's sign*.

SUGGESTED READING AND REFERENCES

1. Oral Radiology—Principles and Interpretation : White and Pharoah, 5th edition.
2. Essentials of Dental Radiography and Radiology. Eric Whaites, 3rd edition.
3. Principles and Practice of Oral Radiographic Interpretations. H.M.Worth.
4. Differential Diagnosis of Oral Lesions. Wood and Goaz.
5. Panoramic Radiology. Langland.

Notes

CHAPTER 12

Developmental Disorders Affecting the Teeth

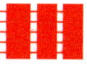

The process of development of a tooth from a tooth bud is complex and involves steps such as histodifferentiation and morphodifferentiation. Any interference to the normal growth pattern can therefore lead to anomalies during development. These anomalies range from alteration in the tooth size, number, their shape and structure. Some of the commonly encountered developmental defects include:

1. Supernumerary teeth
2. Missing teeth/anodontia
3. Microdontia/macrodontia
4. Fusion
5. Concrescence
6. Gemination
7. Taurodontism
8. Dens in dente
9. Dens evaginatus
10. Dilaceration
11. Amelogenesis imperfecta
12. Dentinogenesis imperfecta
13. Dentine dysplasia
14. Regional odontodysplasia

1. Supernumerary Teeth

(i) These are extra teeth that erupt in the arch or may remain impacted within the bone. They may closely resemble the teeth of the groups to which they belong, e.g. paramolars, premolars.

(ii) They are believed to form from a third tooth bud that arises from the dental lamina near the permanent tooth bud.

(iii) The most common supernumerary tooth is a mesiodens that forms between the two central incisors. It may erupt between the incisors or may remain impacted in the bone (Fig. 12.1).

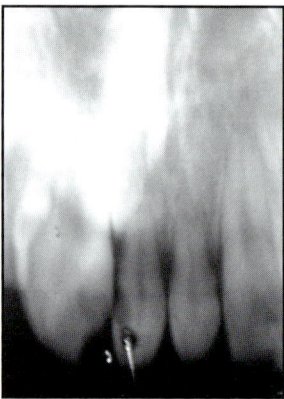

Fig. 12.1: Two mesiodens which have erupted in the arch.

(iv) The next most common tooth is the maxillary fourth molar which if present is often small in size. Supernumerary teeth may occur at any other site, but their occurrence in the deciduous dentition is rare.

(v) Multiple impacted supernumerary teeth may be a feature of cleidocranial dysplasia or Gardner's syndrome.

(vi) Radiographically, they appear as normal appearing tooth often having a different shape.

(vii) They do not pose any significant problems but may sometimes result in malocclusion. If mesiodens is extracted, there is a big diastema, but the space is not enough for aesthetically acceptable restoration. Impacted teeth may undergo cystic changes within the jaws.

(viii) If impacted teeth have to be removed, their position in the jaws must be confirmed by radiographs using the SLOB rule or by identifying their location in a true occlusal view.

2. Missing Tooth/Anodontia

(i) True anodontia refers to congenital absence of teeth. True anodontia may be complete or partial.

(ii) Partial anodontia also known as oligodontia or hypodontia is a more common condition. The most common teeth to remain missing are the third molars followed by the maxillary lateral incisors.

(iii) Anodontia is rare in the deciduous dentition, but if present the most common tooth to be absent is the maxillary lateral incisor.

(iv) Complete anodontia may be a prominent feature of hereditary ectodermal dysplasia which is a genetic condition associated with reduced hair growth in the face and body, absence of sweat glands, defects of the nails, skin and other ectodermal structures (Figs 12.2 and 12.3).

(v) The absence of teeth can be confirmed by obtaining radiographs such as an OPG.

(vi) Once diagnosed, prosthetic rehabilitation must be considered to restore normal function and aesthetics.

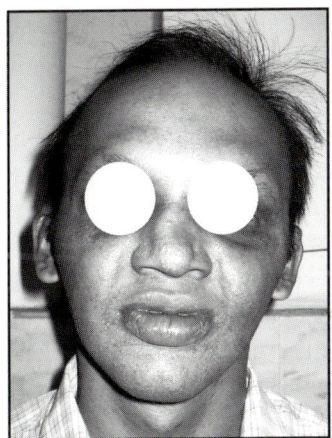

Fig. 12.2: Photograph of a patient with ectodermal dysplasia.

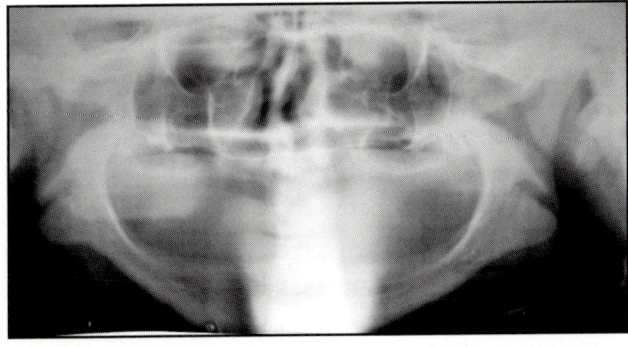

Fig. 12.3: OPG of the same patient showing complete absence of teeth.

3. Microdontia/Macrodontia

  (i) Microdontia is a condition in which the teeth are small in size. Relative microdontia may be present when normal sized teeth are placed in large sized jaws.

 (ii) Generalized microdontia may be a feature of pituitary dwarfism.

(iii) Localized microdontia are commonly found with third molars or peg shape lateral incisors.

(iv) Macrodontia is a condition in which the teeth are large in size. Relative macrodontia may be present when normal sized teeth are placed in small sized jaws.

4. Fusion (Synodontia)

  (i) Fusion is a developmental anomaly that results due to union of two separately formed tooth germs.

 (ii) The main cause of fusion may be the physical force or pressure producing contact between two tooth germs during tooth development.

(iii) If the contact occurs during early stages of development, the two teeth may be completely fused to form a single large tooth, while if it occurs during the later stages, only a portion of their surfaces may be fused.

(iv) Fusion may occur between two normal teeth of the dentition or between a normal and a supernumerary tooth in the arch.

 (v) Radiographically, fused teeth have a large size and show large sized pulp chamber and root canal (Fig. 12.4a).

5. Concrescence

  (i) Concrescence is fusion of teeth by means of cementum alone.

 (ii) It often results because of contact between the roots due to crowding.

(iii) Diagnosis must be made on the basis of radiographic findings where the affected teeth appear to be in contact with their roots. Care must be taken to differentiate this appearance from one that is created because of mere superimposition of roots (Fig. 12.4b).

(iv) Extraction of one of the involved tooth will result in luxation and removal of the adjacent involved tooth, which must be informed to the patient well in advance; else the patient may charge the dentist for negligence.

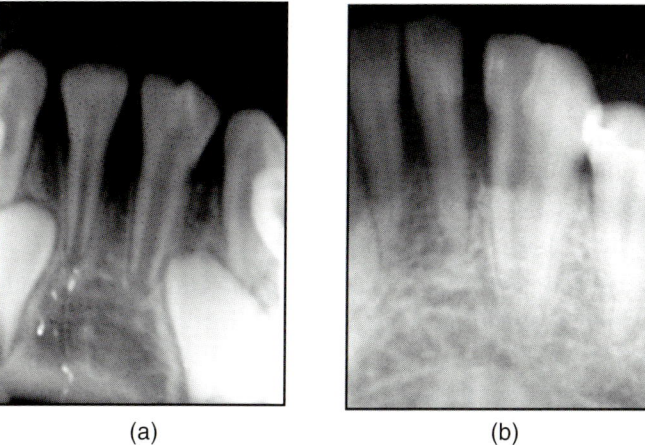

(a)   (b)

Figs 12.4a and b: (a) Fusion of teeth. (b) Concrescence of roots of lateral incisor and canine.

6. Gemination

(i) Gemination is an anomaly which results when the tooth bud attempts to divide by invagination with resultant incomplete formation of two teeth.

(ii) It is also known as twinning.

(iii) Both the dentitions may be affected and the condition is more commonly seen in the incisors.

(iv) Clinically, the crown looks large in size and shows a notch. Radiographically, the altered shape of the pulp chamber and root canal can be noted which may be divided by a partition.

7. Taurodontism

(i) Taurodontism is the name given to a peculiar anomaly in which the body of the tooth is enlarged at the expense of the root. The term literally means bull teeth which are derived due to the similarity in appearance with the teeth of cud chewing animals.

(ii) Taurodontism has been classified into three types: hypotaurodont, mesotaurodont and hypertaurodont, where hypertaurodont represent the most extreme form in which the bifurcation or trifurcation area is very close to the root apex.

(iii) It may be caused due to failure of the Hertwig's epithelial root sheath to invaginate at the correct horizontal level. This condition is heritable and genetically controlled.

(iv) Molars are usually affected, but the teeth appear to be clinically normal.

(v) Radiograph reveals the unusual nature of the teeth which are rectangular instead of a normal conical shape. These teeth have a large pulp chamber that lack the usual constriction at the cervical region (Figs 12.5 and 12.6).

(vi) The roots are short and the furcation area is close to the root apex.

(vii) Taurodontism may be a feature of Klinefelter's syndrome or Down's syndrome.

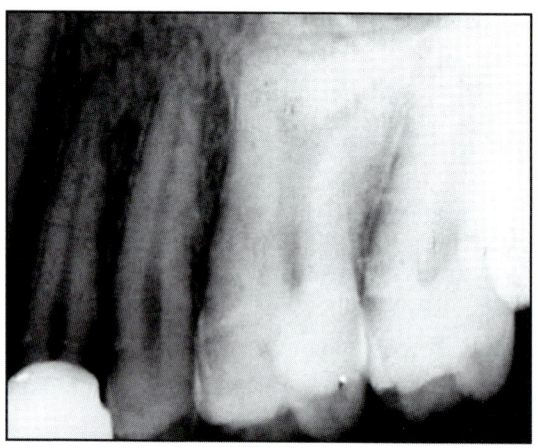

Fig. 12.5: Taurodontism in maxillary first molar.

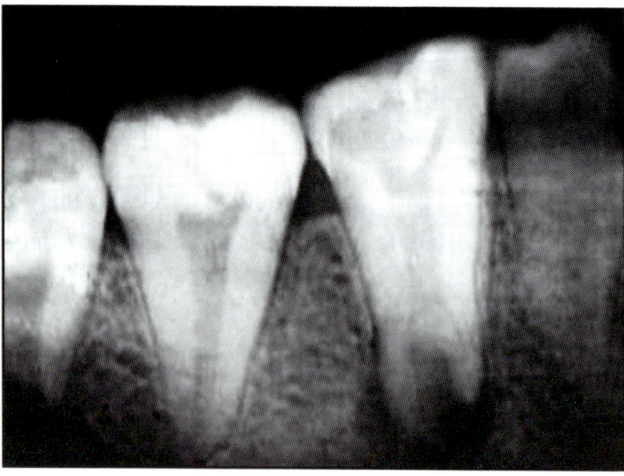

Fig. 12.6: Taurodontism in mandibular first molar.

8. Dens in Dente

(i) Dens in dente also known as dens invaginatus or dilated odontome, is a developmental defect which arises as a result of invagination in the surface of a tooth crown before calcification has occurred. Increased localized external pressure, focal growth retardation and focal growth stimulation in certain areas of the tooth bud may result into such an invagination.

(ii) The most common tooth to be affected is the permanent maxillary lateral incisor. Rarely the premolars may also be affected.

(iii) Dens invaginatus may be of two types, coronal and radicular. The radicular variety forms due to invagination of the Hertwig's epithelial root sheath and is lined by cementum.

(iv) The term dens invaginatus is used when the invagination is from the cingulum of the tooth and the term dens in dente is used to denote invagination from the incisal edge.

(v) Clinically the tooth may be normal in appearance except for a deep lingual pit on the crown and at times it may appear conical and nipple shaped.

(vi) Radiograph shows a tooth in tooth appearance. The affected tooth shows enamel lined tract extending into the pulp chamber and can be clearly seen even before the tooth erupts in the oral cavity (Fig. 12.7).

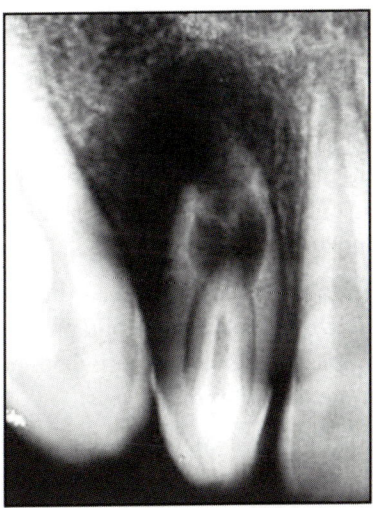

Fig. 12.7: Dens in dente in maxillary lateral incisor.

H.M. Worth has described two more types of dilated odontome.

– A root dilation resembling an open umbrella.

– Fleur-de-lys which resembles the French emblem.

(vii) As the tooth contains an enamel lined tract and the crown has an aperture, there is a free access to microorganisms, food debris, etc. and hence the tooth invariably develops periapical infection very rapidly. At times the canal anatomy is so adversely affected that the affected tooth is not amenable to root canal treatment and has to be extracted to control the infection.

9. Dens Evaginatus

(i) It is also known as Leong's premolar or an evaginated odontome.

(ii) It develops due to proliferation and evagination of an area of inner enamel epithelium and the sub adjacent odontogenic mesenchyme into the dental organ during early tooth development.

(iii) Clinically it is seen as an extra cusp or a globule of enamel on the occlusal surface of the teeth between the buccal and lingual cusps of the premolars.

(iv) They may interfere with complete tooth eruption and can also lead to periapical disease in the absence of caries.

10. Dilaceration

(i) Dilaceration refers to an abnormal curve or bend in the root or crown of the formed teeth.

(ii) Trauma during tooth development can result in the change in the direction of root formation causing an abnormal curvature.

(iii) The curvature may be present in the cervical one third, middle on third or apical one third of the teeth and is evident on the radiograph (Figs 12.8 and 12.9).

(iv) When the curve is in a buccolingual direction, it gives rise to a *bull's eye appearance* on the radiograph as the rays pass through the apical foramen and the surrounding periodontal ligament space which are in the direction of the rays.

(v) Dilacerated teeth pose a challenge during root canal treatment or extraction.

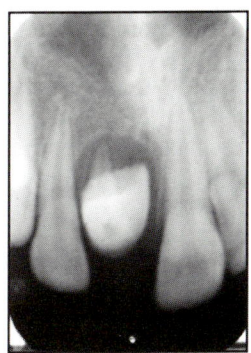

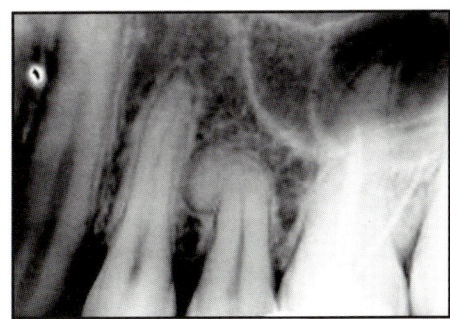

Fig. 12.8: Radiograph of a dilacerated tooth.

Fig. 12.9: Radiograph of a dilacerated root.

11. Amelogenesis Imperfecta

(i) Amelogenesis imperfecta is an autosomal dominant or X-linked disorder affecting the teeth.

(ii) The enamel forms through the stages of matrix formation, calcification and maturation. Depending upon the stage at which the defect takes place, the following types have been identified.

(a) Hypoplastic

(b) Hypocalcification

(c) Hypomaturation

(d) Hypocalcification/hypomaturation—combination type.

(iii) In the hypoplastic variety, the enamel fails to develop to its normal thickness. Hence, the underlying dentine is seen through and the tooth acquires a yellowish brown colour. The surface of the crown may appear smooth or pitted in certain areas. In some varieties, the entire crown may have a pitted appearance, while the agenesis type may show total absence of enamel.

(iv) The hypomaturation type has a normal enamel thickness, but the surface is mottled. The enamel is softer and chips off easily with a probe. The teeth appear as if they are snow capped with zone of opaque enamel on the incisal edges and cusp tips.

(v) The hypocalcified type is more common and the enamel and dentine are soft, which are soon lost after eruption. Severe attrition of the crown results in the crown being reduced to the gingival level. The crowns appear dark and get stained quickly.

(vi) The combination type shows features of both hypoplastic and hypomaturative types.

(vii) Radiographic appearance (Fig. 12.10)

(a) The hypoplastic type appears as square-shaped teeth with thin opaque enamel and low or absent cusps. Pitting of the crown is seen as localized areas of reduced density on the crown.

(b) In the hypomaturative type, the enamel thickness is normal but the density of enamel is same as that of dentine.

(c) In the hypocalcified type, the enamel density is less than that of the dentine. Obliteration of the pulp chamber may also be present.

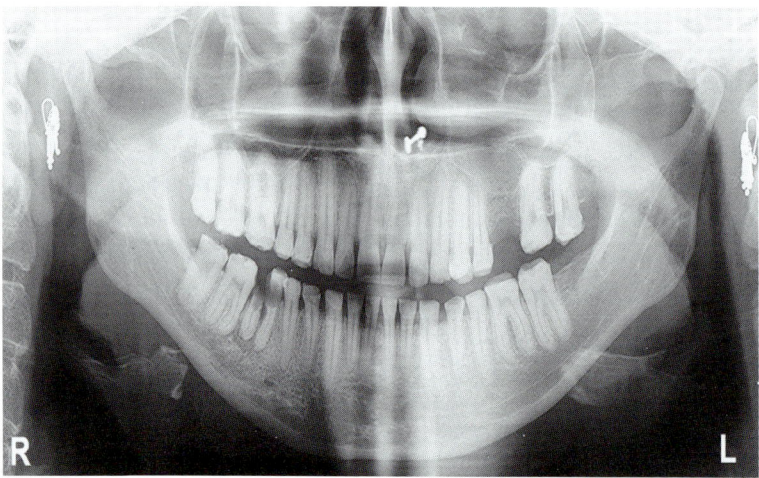

Fig. 12.10: OPG showing amelogenesis imperfecta affecting all the teeth.

12. Dentinogenesis Imperfecta

(i) Also known as hereditary opalescent dentine, it is primarily a disorder of dentine affecting the enamel secondarily. It is an autosomal dominant disease affecting both sexes equally.

(ii) Three types of dentinogenesis imperfecta have been identified:

Type I : Dentinogenesis imperfecta associated with osteogenesis imperfecta.

Type II : Dentinogenesis imperfecta not associated with osteogenesis imperfecta.

Type III : Brandy wine type.

(iii) The crowns of the teeth appear as amber-like translucency with colour varying from blue to light yellow.

(iv) The enamel easily fractures and the teeth may easily wear down till the level of gingiva. Anterior open bite is usually present.

(v) Radiographically, the teeth appear as having a bulbous crown with a marked constriction at the cervix. Mild to marked attrition of the incisal edges and occlusal surfaces is noted (Fig.10.11).

(vi) In the type I and II cases, the pulp chambers may be partially or completely obliterated. Type III cases have large pulp chambers and appear as shell teeth.

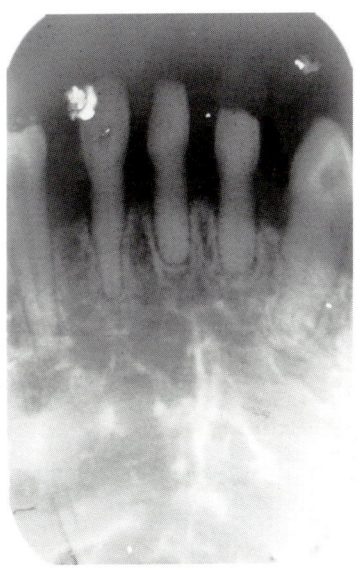

Fig. 12.11: Teeth affected by dentinogenesis imperfecta.

13. Dentin Dysplasia

(i) It is an autosomal dominant trait that resembles dentinogenesis imperfecta.

(ii) Two types have been identified:

Type I : Radicular

Type II : Coronal

(iii) Cases of type I dentin dysplasia may appear normal clinically, but are often misaligned. The roots are short and the pulp chamber may be completely obliterated before eruption of teeth. These teeth may show periapical radiolucencies which may be cysts or granulomas.

(iv) The type II cases appear similar to dentinogenesis imperfecta. The root length is normal. The teeth have normal sized pulp chamber at the time of eruption which may get obliterated later on. The pulp chambers eventually acquire a flame shape or a thistle tube like shape and may contain many pulp stones (Fig. 12.12).

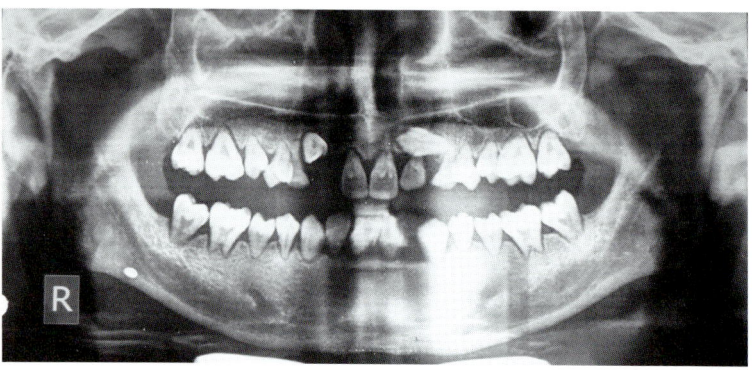

Fig. 12.12: OPG showing dentin dysplasia.

14. Regional Odontodysplasia (Ghost teeth/Odontogenesis imperfecta)

(i) This is a non hereditary condition which affects both enamel and dentine.

(ii) Alteration in the vascularity to the tooth buds; local trauma, infection, etc. are known to be the causative factor.

(iii) One or more teeth are involved in a given region and the teeth are stained brown and exhibit mottling.

(iv) Many of these teeth may fail to erupt, but if they erupt, they are quickly affected by caries or periodontal disease.

(v) Radiographically, extremely thin enamel and dentine is seen surrounding a large pulp space. The teeth thus have a pale wispy image and are therefore referred to as *Ghost teeth*. The root outlines are short and ill-defined with open apices. The enlarged pulp chamber may have one or more pulp stones in them (Fig. 12.13).

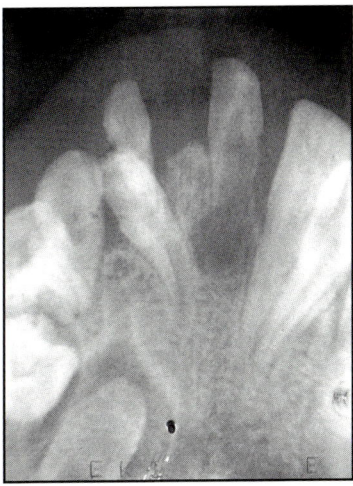

Fig. 12.13: Radiograph showing regional odontodysplasia.

SUGGESTED READING AND REFERENCES

1. Oral Radiology—Principles and Interpretation: White and Pharoah 5th edition.
2. Essentials of Dental Radiography and Radiology—Eric Whaites, 3rd edition.
3. Principles and Practice of Oral Radiographic Interpretations—H.M.Worth.
4. Differential Diagnosis of Oral Lesions—Wood and Goaz.
5. Oral and Maxillofacial Pathology, 2nd edition—Neville.
6. A Textbook of Oral Pathology, Shafer, 4th edition.

Notes

CHAPTER 13

Salivary Gland Diseases

The main source of saliva in the mouth is from the three pairs of major salivary glands namely the parotid, submandibular and the sublingual glands. The minor salivary glands are distributed throughout the submucosa in the oral cavity and also secrete saliva, thereby contributing to the volume of whole saliva. The total saliva produced per day is about 1 to 1.5 liters. Out of this 60% is produced by the parotid, 30% by the submandibular gland, 5% is contributed by the sublingual gland and the remaining 5% comes from the minor salivary glands. The normal salivary flow rate is 0.05 ml per minute.

The whole saliva obtained from the mouth is a composite of saliva secreted from the individual glands, the gingival crevicular fluid and also contains epithelial cells, microbes and debris.

Composition of Saliva

1. Saliva is a colourless, slightly alkaline fluid with a pH of 6.4 to 7.1. It contains 99% or more of water and 0.6% solids. Out of this 0.2% is made of organic and 0.4% of inorganic constituents.

2. The major salivary electrolytes are Na^+, K^+, Cl^-, and HCO_3^-. Other trace elements include Ca^{2+}, Mg^{2+}, SCN^- (thiocyanate) and F^-.

3. **Non electrolytes:** Urea and uric acids are present in the saliva which are derived from the blood. The saliva is low in protein content. Glycoproteins such as mucin are present in the saliva which provide viscosity to saliva.

4. **Salivary amylase:** It is a digestive enzyme present mainly in the parotid saliva that helps in the digestion of starch. Submandibular gland secretes only 20% of amylase, while sublingual and the minor salivary glands do not produce it since they have no serous components.

5. **Secretory IgA:** Immunoglobulin A (SIgA) is present in the saliva, which contributes to the antiviral and antibacterial actions of saliva. Trace amount of IgM and IgG are also present.

6. Antibacterial agents such as lysozymes, lactoperoxidase and thiocyanate are also present in saliva.

Functions of Saliva

1. **Lubrication and protection of mucous membrane:** The glycoproteins line the oral mucosa providing barrier against potential harmful agents.

2. **Mechanical cleansing:** Saliva acts as a backward tide to remove the food and debris. Thereby it provides protection against caries and periodontal disease.

3. **Maintenance of tooth integrity:** The salivary salts allow post eruptive maturation, thereby preventing dissolution of tooth structure. A film of glycoprotein covers the tooth structure that reduces the effects of wear and tear on the tooth.

4. **Buffering action:** HCO_3^- and PO_4^- ions present in the saliva help to buffer the sugar derived acidity in the saliva.

5. **Digestive action:** The salivary amylase present in the saliva brings about the digestion of carbohydrates by converting them to maltose. This activity of amylase takes place for 30 minutes after the food reaches the stomach before being inactivated by the acids in the stomach.

Classification of Salivary Gland Diseases

The diseases affecting salivary glands can be classified as follows:

I. Developmental anomalies

(i) Aplasia of the gland

(ii) Hypoplasia of the gland

(iii) Aberrant salivary gland

(iv) Accessory salivary ducts

(v) Diverticuli in salivary duct

(vi) Atresia of the ducts

II. Functional disorders of salivary glands

(i) Increased salivary secretion – Sialorrhea/Ptyalism

(ii) Reduced salivary secretion – Xerostomia

III. Inflammatory disorders
(i) Viral sialoadenitis—Mumps
(ii) Bacterial sialoadenitis
(iii) Allergic sialoadenitis
(iv) Necrotising sialometaplasia

IV. Obstructive salivary gland disorders
(i) Sialolithiasis
(ii) Mucocele—Mucous retention/extravasation cyst
(iii) Ranula

V Sialadenosis:
It is the non inflammatory, non neoplastic asymptomatic salivary gland enlargement which may be due to metabolic, endocrine or drug induced causes

VI. Autoimmune diseases
(i) Sjögren's syndrome
(ii) Mickulicz's disease

VII. Salivary gland neoplasms

A. Benign tumors
(i) Pleomorphic adenoma
(ii) Monomorphic adenoma
(iii) Papillary cyst adenoma lymphomatosum (Warthin's tumor)

B. Malignant tumors
(i) Adenoid cystic carcinoma
(ii) Mucoepidermoid carcinoma
(iii) Carcinoma ex pleomorphic adenoma

IMAGING MODALITIES FOR SALIVARY GLAND DISEASES

The various imaging modalities to study the salivary glands are as follows:

1. PLAIN FILM RADIOGRAPHY

Plain films are used to study stones in the salivary glands. The parotid glands can be studied with OPG, lateral oblique view, AP view. An IOPA film can be placed in the buccal sulcus in the parotid papilla region and exposed to study stones in the Stenson's duct. The submandibular salivary glands can be studied with true occlusal view of the mandible, OPG or a lateral oblique view.

2. SIALOGRAPHY

Sialography is one of the oldest modality to study the ductal system of the salivary glands described by Carpy in 1902. It is a technique in which a radiopaque dye is injected into the ducts of the gland and a radiographic image is obtained.

Indications of Sialography

Sialography is indicated in the following cases:

 (i) To study sialoliths that are radiolucent.
 (ii) To study the extent of destruction of the duct caused by a sialolith or a foreign body.
 (iii) To study and diagnose fistulas and diverticuli.
 (iv) To study recurrent inflammations of the salivary glands.
 (v) To demonstrate a tumor, its location, extent and size.
 (vi) To outline the plane of facial nerve before obtaining biopsies.
 (vii) Therapeutic dilatation of strictures by forceful injection of the dye.

The contraindications of sialography include:

 (i) Patients who are allergic to contrast media.
 (ii) Acute infections of salivary glands, as the ductal lining becomes thin and may rupture during sialography. The infection may be pushed deeper down into the gland during sialography.
 (iii) Patients who are scheduled to undergo thyroid function test because the iodine present in the dye interferes with thyroid functioning.

Contrast Media

Two main types of contrast media are available, water soluble and oil based.

The water soluble dyes fill the fine ductules and require low injection pressure. Also if they are accidentally extravasated, they are absorbed by the body and do not trigger any foreign body reaction, e.g. hypaque, renograffin.

The fat soluble agents provide excellent opacification of ducts, but they require high injection pressure and can evoke a foreign body reaction if extravasated, e.g. ethiodol, lipodiol.

Armamentarium for Sialography

The instruments and materials required to perform a successful sialography are a cannula, lacrimal dilator, rubber tubing, syringes 5–10 cc, contrast medium, lemon slices, X-ray films and cassettes.

Steps in Sialography

1. **Clinical examination**

   A detailed clinical examination must be performed to identify the various features of the disease.

2. **Preliminary radiographic examination**

   If an osteolytic lesion is seen on the ramus in patients with salivary gland swellings, it is suggestive of malignancy.

   A plain film radiographic survey must be made to ascertain the presence of any radiopaque masses in the salivary glands. Appropriate views must be obtained to study the gland under question completely.

3. **Cannulation of the duct**

   The ductal orifices are identified by drying the area and milking the gland, appearance of a drop of saliva helps to locate the orifice. The duct is then cannulated successfully to allow the dye to be injected into the gland. The cannula must not be forced into the duct if any resistance is encountered as this may traumatize the duct and cause extravasation of the dye. This is called as iatrogenic pseudoduct formation.

4. **Injection of the contrast medium**

   The hand injection method using a needle and syringe is the preferred method. About 0.5 to 0.75 cc of the dye is injected into the parotid gland, while 0.5 cc is injected into the submandibular gland.

5. **Phases of sialography**

   (a) **Ductal phase:** This phase begins with the injection of the dye until the parenchyma begins to appear. The parotid ductal anatomy is uniform with progressive arborization (branching) giving it a leafless tree like appearance. The submandibular ductal system shows non uniform arborization with the terminal duct terminating abruptly.

(b) **Acinar phase:** This phase begins with the increase in the overall density of the gland and can be used to study the parenchymal pattern.

(c) **Evacuation phase:** A radiograph is obtained in the post evacuation phase to study the retention of dye within the gland as it may occur in siaolithiasis and strictures of the gland.

A normal Sialogram (Fig. 13.1)

In a normal sialogram, the Stenson's duct measures about 6–8 cm in length, 1–3 mm in diameter, located 2 mm lateral to the ramus of the mandible (in lateral views), fine with uniform arborization.

The submandibular gland duct has two portions, the superficial and the deep parts with the coma-shaped area joining them. The duct measures 5 cm in length, 2–4 mm wide with a narrow orifice and there is abrupt ending of the secondary ducts.

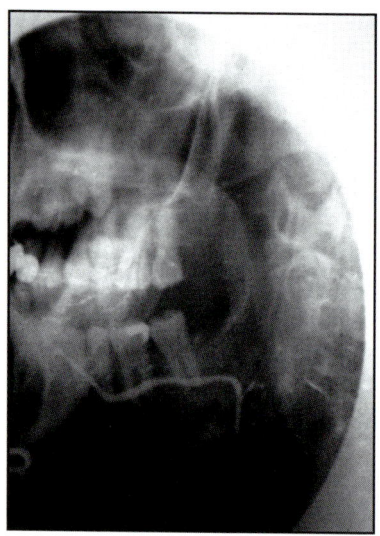

Fig. 13.1: Normal sialogram of the submandibular gland.

Sialographic Appearance in Various Diseases

(i) *Sialoliths: Filling defect* with segmental strictures and retention of the contrast medium are seen on a sialogram (Fig. 13.2).

(ii) *Sialodochitis*: Segmental stricture of the duct gives rise to a *sausage string* appearance of the duct (Fig. 13.3).

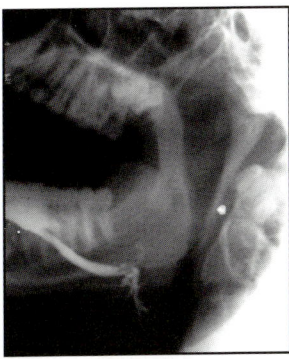

Fig. 13.2: Sialogram showing a filling defect at the coma area.

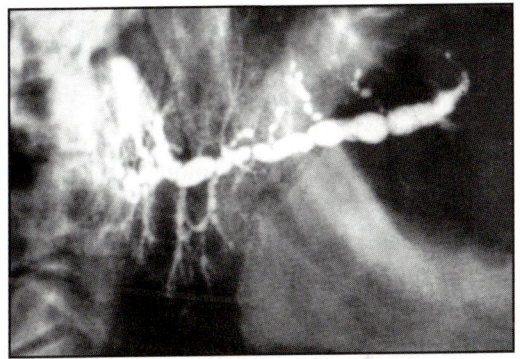

Fig. 13.3: Sialogram showing sausage string appearance in sialodochitis.

(iii) *Sialadenitis*: Terminal ectasia (dilatation) is seen with an *apple tree* like appearance.

(iv) *Sjögren's syndrome*: Acinar ectasia giving rise to *cherry blossom* appearance is seen (Fig. 13.4).

(v) *Benign tumors*: Splaying of ducts giving rise to *ball in hand appearance* (Fig. 13.5).

(vi) *Ductal* irregularity with abnormal contrast puddling on a sialogram is suggestive of a malignant tumor of the salivary gland.

(vii) *The 18 mm rule*: If in an AP parotid sialogram, the duct is displaced more than 18 mm from the ramus, it is an indication of presence of a mass within the gland. Exception to this rule is the presence of masseteric hypertrophy (Fig. 13.5).

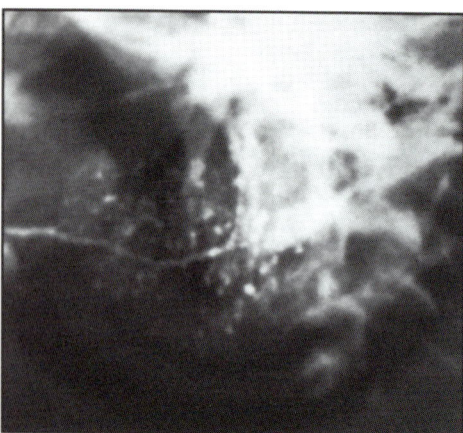

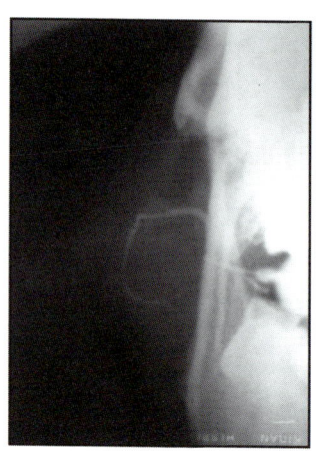

Fig. 13.4: A sialogram showing cherry blossom appearance.

Fig. 13.5: A parotid sialogram showing ball in hand appearance.

3. RADIONUCLIDE SCANNING/SCINTIGRAPHY

Technetium pertechtenate 99 m, a radioisotope is taken up by the salivary gland after intravenous injection and transported through the glands to be secreted by the ducts. This forms the basis of radionuclide scanning which is used to detect the functioning of the tissues. The main indications of salivary scintigraphy are:

(i) Ductal obstruction/sialoliths, i.e. when sialography cannot be performed.

(ii) To study salivary gland aplasia.

(iii) To study salivary gland tumors.

(iv) To study and diagnose Sjögren's syndrome.

Technique

10–20 mCi of ^{99m}Tc is injected intravenously. The uptake, concentration and washout phases are imaged using a gamma camera and studied on a scintigram.

(a) *Flow phase:* It lasts for 15–20 seconds after injecting the radiopharmaceutical agent and represents the phase where the dye is distributed in the body and the gland.

(b) *Concentration phase*: This is the phase during which the tracer steadily begins to concentrate within the gland and rises in 10 minutes. In a normal salivary scintigram, the tracer shows uniform symmetrical uptake of the tracer.

(c) *Wash out phase*: This phase represents the evacuation of tracer from the gland. A normal gland must clear promptly, uniformly and symmetrically.

In most cases of salivary gland disease, the tracer does not concentrate in the gland except in cases of Warthin's tumor and Oncocytoma which appear as hot-spots in a scintigram because these tumors do not communicate with the ductal system and cause retention of the tracer.

4. CT SCANS

The parotid gland appears as a triangular shaped gland located posterolateral to the mandible between the masseter and the sternocleidomastoid. It is predominantly composed of fibro-fatty tissue and hence has a low CT number (-10 to 10 HU). Thus it appears as a slightly hypodense mass on the CT and also enhances on contrast administration with its CT number increasing up to 10–20 HU. The submandibular gland is an L-shaped gland divided into superficial and deep lobes by the mylohyoid muscle. As compared to the parotid, it has a higher CT density of about 35–60 HU. CT scans are valuable in the diagnosis of sialoliths, benign and malignant tumors of salivary gland, infections and abscess cavities within the gland.

5. MRI SCANS

In a normal MRI scan, the salivary glands appear as soft tissue densities slightly greater in intensity than muscle but lesser than fat. MRI can be used to study tumors involving the salivary glands and Sjögren's syndrome.

6. ULTRASONOGRAPHY

USG can be used to study sialoliths, cyst and tumors within the salivary gland. The deep lobe of parotid cannot be studied with a USG since it underlies the thick bone of the ramus of the mandible. USG can also be used to guide biopsy and FNAC procedures.

DEVELOPMENTAL ANOMALIES

ABERRANT/ECTOPIC SALIVARY GLAND

Salivary gland may develop at unusual sites apart from the oral cavity. The most common sites include the neck, posterior part of the mandible or the condyles. Such aberrant gland must not be mistaken for minor salivary glands or other diseases. A sialography or biopsy may be helpful to identify the gland in such cases.

Aplasia/Hypoplasia

Aplasia of major salivary glands is a rare occurrence. If present, it may be associated with cleft palate or mandibulofacial dysostosis. Hypoplasia of salivary gland may be associated with Melkerson-Rosenthal syndrome which also shows features such as fissured tongue, facial palsy, orofacial granulomatosis. The absence of saliva in the mouth is of clinical significance in such cases.

Accessory Salivary Gland Ducts

Extra ducts may be present which either join the main duct or may open separately in the oral cavity.

Diverticuli

Diverticuli are out pockets of the ductal system which may lead to stagnation of saliva resulting in repeated episodes of parotitis. A sialography can be performed to diagnose diverticuli.

Atresia of salivary ducts is a rare finding in which there is congenital absence or occlusion of major salivary gland ducts. It may result in the formation of a retention cyst or produce xerostomia.

Functional Disorders Affecting the Salivary Glands

Sialorrhea

Sialorrhea refers to increased salivation. The causes of sialorrhea include:

1. *Physiologic causes:*
   (a) Infancy
   (b) During eruption of teeth
   (c) Starvation
   (d) Insertion of new dentures or oral appliances
2. *Pathologic causes:*
   (a) Local mouth diseases: ANUG, erythema multiforme, metal poisoning.
   (b) Systemic diseases: Mental retardation, epilepsy, facial paralysis, alcoholic neuritis, parkinsonism, morphine addiction, etc.
   (c) Drugs: Pilocarpine (due to stimulation of CNS), potassium iodide, mercurial salts (by causing irritation to the gland).

Clinical Features and Management

1. Saliva constantly drools from the mouth which also causes social embarrassment to the patient. In conditions such as parkinsonism, drooling of saliva may be due to the impaired neuromuscular control rather the excess production of saliva.

2. Frequent drooling of saliva keeps the corners of the mouth moist thereby predisposing to candidiasis and angular cheilitis and skin infection.

While managing these patients, the exact cause of sialorrhea must be identified. If it is because of systemic causes, they must be treated accordingly. Anti-sialagogue such as belladonna alkaloids (atropine) can be given to the patient to control salivary production. Probanthin (Propantheline) is a anti-cholinergic drug that can help to reduce salivary secretion.

Xerostomia (Asialorrhea)

Xerostomia refers to reduced salivary production resulting in dry mouth.

The causes of xerostomia are:

1. Diseases of salivary glands, e.g. aplasia/hypoplasia, ductal obstruction, irradiation to salivary glands.

2. Drugs – Many drugs are implicated in the occurrence of xerostomia. Notable ones include anti histaminic, anti cholinergic such as atropine, tricyclic antidepressants, anti parkinsonism drugs, anti hypertensive drugs.

3. Systemic diseases like fever, dehydration, lung infections, typhoid, uncontrolled diabetes, hyperthyroidism, vitamin A and B complex deficiency, etc. can result in reduced salivary secretion.

4. Physiological causes – menopause.

5. Occupational exposure to organic dust and zinc poisoning.

6. Psychological causes – Fear and anxiety.

7. Sjögren's syndrome.

Clinical Features and Management

(a) The patient complains of dryness in the mouth, burning sensation, difficulty in eating and speech.

(b) On examination, the mouth appears dry with the lips sticking to each other.

(c) The mucosa may be pale, dry and erythematous. Cracks and fissures my be present on the mucosa.

(d) Patients who have undergone radiation therapy can also have significant xerostomia accompanied with radiation caries.

(e) Symptomatic treatment may be provided by increasing the fluid intake, frequent sipping of water and use of artificial saliva (*wet mouth*).

(f) Moisturizing agents such as cold cream or paraffin oil or vaseline can be applied to the lips for symptomatic relief.

(g) Secretagogues such as orange or lemon candy can be used to stimulate saliva. However, sugarless candies are recommended to prevent dental caries.

(h) Sialagogue drugs such as Pilocarpine, Bromhexine, Cevimiline and Anetholetrithione have been tried in the management of xerostomia.

INFLAMMATORY DISORDERS

Mumps

1. Mumps is an acute contagious viral infection characterized by bilateral salivary gland enlargement, usually the parotid. It is a disease of childhood and rarely affects elders where it has a greater tendency to develop complications.

2. Mumps is caused by paramyxovirus which is an RNA virus and has an incubation period of 3 weeks. The condition can occur in epidemics.

3. A firm tender swelling of the parotid gland appears around the ear causing the ear lobule to be raised (unlike the third molar swelling). Mouth opening becomes painful and restricted.

4. Systemic symptoms such as fever, malaise and anorexia may be present.

5. The opening of the parotid duct or the papilla may appear puffy and reddened.

Management of Mumps

(i) Symptomatic treatment must be provided to the patient with anti inflammatory and anti pyretic drugs.

(ii) The condition is usually self-limiting, but occasionally gives rise to complication. Involvement of testis and ovaries (orchitis and oophoritis respectively) can result in sterility.

The other organs to be affected are the pancreas, myocardium, mammary glands, etc.

(iii) Systemic corticosteroids are indicated when mumps is complicated by painful testicular involvement.

(iv) Mumps can be prevented by vaccinating the child with the MMR (Measles Mumps Rubella) vaccine at the age of 9 months.

Acute Bacterial Sialoadenitis

1. Acute bacterial sialoadenitis is an infectious disease commonly seen in debilitated and dehydrated patients who have undergone surgical procedures. Hence it is also called as surgical parotitis. Due to reduced salivary flow, there is retrograde progression of infection through the salivary ducts resulting in frank pus formation inside the glands. The serous nature of the parotid secretion does not obstruct the ingress of organisms (unlike viscous secretions).

2. A tender, warm swelling with a reddened skin is a presenting feature and pus can be seen dribbling from the Stenson's duct opening in the mouth.

3. Sialography is contraindicated because the disrupted ductal system may rupture allowing the contrast medium to extravasate and evoke a foreign body reaction.

4. If an abscess cavity is present, it can be demonstrated on a CT, USG or MRI scan.

5. Treatment includes antibiotic therapy after culture and sensitivity tests and surgical drainage in some cases.

6. Fluid and electrolyte balance must be maintained and salivary production may be stimulated by asking the patient to suck on lemon candy.

Necrotizing Sialometaplasia

1. It is a benign inflammatory disease affecting the salivary gland tissue that clinically and histologically resembles malignancy. Local ischemia resulting in acinar necrosis is the cause of this disease.

2. Men in their third and fourth decades of life are most commonly affected. The minor salivary glands of the palate are the most common location to be involved where the lesion presents as an ulcer.

3. The lesions have a sudden onset and appear as a nodule which quickly ruptures to form ulcers. The ulcers are often large but painless.

4. Lesion is self-limiting and heals with secondary intention. Debridement of the ulcer and saline mouth rinses will help to fasten the healing process.

Obstructive Salivary Gland Disorders

Sialolithiasis

It is the formation of hard calcified mass within the duct of the salivary gland.

Etiology

1. Inflammatory conditions of the gland, anti cholinergic medications or irregularities in the salivary duct result in pooling of saliva within the duct that encourages stone formation.

2. Calcification may occur around a central nidus within the duct causing stone formation. This central nidus may be a foreign body, microbes within the gland or destroyed epithelial cells.

3. An altered salivary pH, abnormal serum calcium and phosphorus levels also play an important role in a sialolith formation.

4. Thus the pre-requisites for formation of a sialolith are, a neurohormonal condition that causes stagnation of saliva, a central nidus, a metabolic mechanism favoring precipitation of salts.

Composition of Stones

The stones are mainly composed of calcium salts ($CaPO_4$). Traces of magnesium, ammonia are also present. The organic matrix is made up of carbohydrates and amino acids.

The stones formed in the major salivary glands are round, ovoid or elongated and measure a few mm to 2 cm in diameter. Minor salivary gland stones are arranged as large well organized mass or multiple small aggregates.

Sites of Sialolith Formation

The most common site for sialolith formation is the submandibular gland where 80% of the stones are found. Parotid gland accounts to 19% and sublingual gland 1% of the sialoliths formed in the major salivary glands.

The minor salivary glands of the upper lip and buccal mucosa are also rare sites of salivary stone formation.

The reasons why sialoliths are most common in the submandibular glands are as follows:

- (i) Viscous nature of the submandibular saliva due to mucoid secretion.
- (ii) Tortuous course of the duct and takes a right angled bend behind the mylohyoid muscle (the coma area).
- (iii) The orifice of the duct is smaller and its lumen is larger in diameter.
- (iv) The orifice is at a higher level than the gland. This causes stagnation of saliva as it has to move against the gravity.
- (v) Frequent exposure of the duct to trauma.
- (vi) Possible irritation of the papilla by dental calculus.
- (vii) Presence of diverticula which results in stasis.
- (viii) Constriction of the duct caused by the lingual nerve.

The most common location of stone formation in the submandibular duct is the coma-shaped area where the duct crosses the posterior border of the mylohyoid muscle and in the parotid gland is the area before the hilum and the anterior border of masseter where the duct takes a 90° turn.

Clinical Features

1. The most common presenting symptom is recurrent painful enlargement of the gland. The pain and swelling increases with intake of food and subside after a while.
2. In chronic cases, the symptoms may be severe and continuous and may not have any relation to intake of food.
3. The affected gland is tender and enlarged with the overlying skin usually warm and inflamed.
4. Salivary production from the affected duct may be diminished.
5. When the sialolith is present superficially in the duct, it can be palpated and small stones can be milked out of the duct to provide relief to the patients (Figs 13.6a and b).

Radiographic Findings

Plain film radiographs with less exposure are first made to ascertain the presence of calculus. The appearance of calculi on plain film depends upon the degree of calcification, exposure factor and type of projection used. Only 50–70% parotid sialoliths are radiopaque. 80–90% submandibular

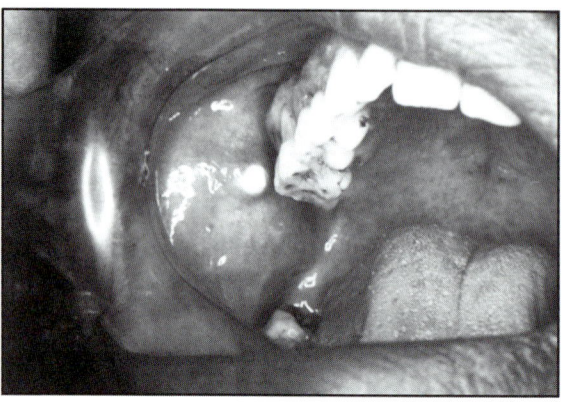

Fig. 13.6a: A superficial sialolith present near the opening of the Stenson's duct.

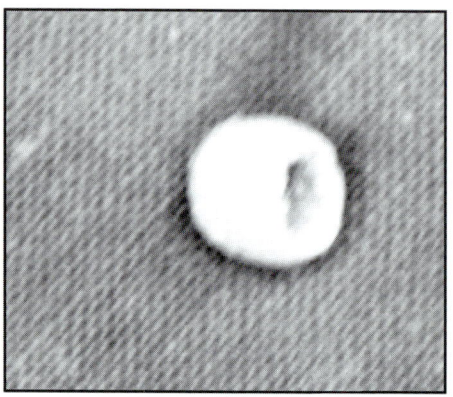

Fig. 13.6b: The sialolith which was recovered from the duct in the above case.

sialolith are radiopaque and the remaining ones are poorly calcified and cannot be seen on the radiograph (Figs 13.7 and 13.8).

The frequently recommended views are mandibular true occlusal, Donavan's technique; 15° lateral oblique, OPG, AP view and intraoral view with an IOPA film placed on the buccal mucosa.

Sialography is a valuable tool to diagnose radiolucent calculi which appear as filling defect with the dye flowing around the stone (Fig. 13.2).

CT scans are highly sensitive in detecting calcified masses within the salivary gland. USG also aids in identifying and localizing sialoliths. Sialoliths appear as echodense (white) spots with acoustic shadow on the USG (Fig. 13.9).

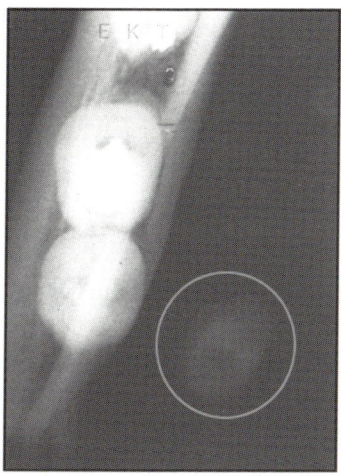

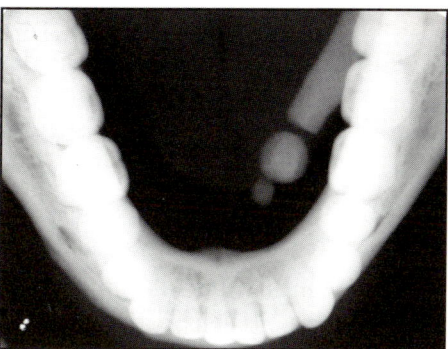

Fig. 13.8: Occlusal view showing large sialolith in the submandibular gland duct.

Fig. 13.7: Occlusal view showing a sialolith in the submandibular gland duct.

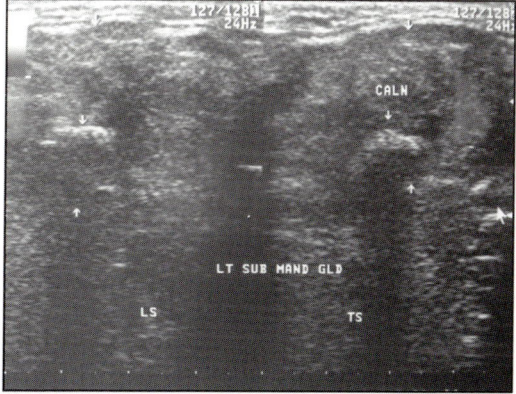

Fig. 13.9: USG showing salivary calculus (caln) in the left submandibular gland.

D.D.   Calcified lymph node
         Foreign body/Avulsed tooth
         Phlebolith
         Tonsillolith
         Myositis ossificans
         Calcified facial artery

Management of Sialolithiasis

(a) Conservative methods include massaging the gland to remove the stones, use of sialogogues to stimulate salivary secretion (Vitamin C chewable tablets) are helpful in removing small stones from the duct and providing relief to the patient.

(b) If the stones are large and located within the duct, surgical methods like sialolithotomy or sialadenectomy must be performed.

(c) Stones within the minor salivary gland can be removed by excisional biopsy.

(d) Lithotripsy is a new method of treating salivary stones where fragmentation of stones is achieved by using shock waves.

Complications of sialoliths include acute suppurative abscess, sinus tract formation, ductal ulceration, stricture formation, progressive pressure atrophy of glandular acini and glandular fibrosis.

Mucocele

1. They are soft cystic swellings caused due to accumulation of saliva within a traumatized or an obstructed duct.

2. The extravasations are seen frequently on the lips, buccal mucosa and retromolar area and not lined by any epithelial lining. Mucous retention phenomena are seen often on the hard palate and floor of the mouth and caused due to ductal obstruction by sialolith or strictures.

3. They appear as well-defined, soft, smooth fluctuant swelling with a typical blue hue.

4. Surgical removal is the treatment of choice and recurrences are common due to the adjacent minor salivary gland getting traumatized during surgery.

Ranula

1. Ranulas are large mucoceles formed in the floor of the mouth. They are often associated with the sublingual duct and may be caused by a retention or extravasation phenomenon.

2. They present as slow growing, soft and fluctuant swelling in the floor of the mouth having a blue color that resembles the belly of a frog. Hence, they are named as ranula.

3. Deeper lesions may herniate through the mylohyoid muscle and extend into the neck. They are called as plunging ranula.

4. Surgical removal or marsupialization is the treatment of choice.

SJÖGREN'S SYNDROME

Sjögren's syndrome (Sicca syndrome) is an autoimmune disorder affecting the exocrine glands and may be associated with connective tissue disease, neuropathy and lymphoproliferative disorders. Primary Sjögren's syndrome is a disease that affects only the lacrimal and salivary glands. Secondary Sjögren's syndrome is also associated connective tissue disorders like rheumatoid arthritis, polymyositis, systemic lupus erythematosus, scleroderma, etc.

Clinical Features

1. This disease has a predilection for post menopausal women and is about 9 times more common in females than males.

2. Dryness in the mouth causing difficulty in eating and speech is the presenting symptom. Patients also complain of dryness in the eye, throat and nose.

3. Patients who are wearing dentures are unable to retain the dentures and suffer from recurrent oral ulcers and candidiasis. They also feel the need to sip water frequently.

4. The normal pooling of saliva is absent in the mouth and the lips stick to each other. When a tongue blade is used to retract the tongue or cheeks, it sticks to the mucosa.

5. Patients may have dried and cracked lips and are more vulnerable to dental caries.

Diagnosis of Sjögren's Syndrome

Sialography

Sialographic studies may show presence of punctate, globular or cavitary pseudo sialectases within the gland which are filled with radiopaque dye. These are called as pseudo sialectases as these appear because of extravasation of the dye and not because of dilatation of the ductules. This appearance is called as *branchless fruit laden tree appearance* or *cherry blossom appearance* (Fig. 13.4).

MRI scans can be used to differentiate between swelling of glands due to Sjögren's syndrome and other pathologies. A salt and pepper appearance on the MRI scan is highly suggestive of Sjögren's syndrome.

Scintigraphy

Scintigraphic studies with technetium pertechtenate shows delayed appearance of tracer in the oral cavity due to reduced salivary secretion.

Minor salivary gland biopsy for diagnosis of Sjögren's syndrome.

Minor salivary gland biopsy (usually from the lips) shows diffuse infiltration of lymphocytes within the glandular parenchyma destroying it. A grading system has been formulated for the diagnosis of Sjögren's syndrome based upon the minor salivary gland biopsy findings which is as follows:

  (i) The number of infiltrating mononuclear cells are determined and an aggregate of 50 or more is termed as one focus.

 (ii) The number of such foci and the total area in which they were found are measured.

(iii) The number of such foci per 4 sq mm area is calculated and called as focus score which ranges from 0 to 12.

(iv) A focus score of more than 1 is considered to be suggestive of Sjögren's syndrome.

San Diego diagnostic criteria for Sjögren's syndrome

  I. Primary Sjögren's syndrome

   A. Ocular dryness

   1. Schirmmer's lacrimal test showing less than 8 mm of wetting in 5 minutes.

      AND

   2. Positive Rose Bengal staining to demonstrate keratoconjunctivitis sicca.

   B. Symptoms and signs of oral dryness

   1. Reduced parotid flow demonstrated using Lashley's cup or other methods.

      AND

   2. Abnormal biopsy of minor salivary gland with a focus score more than or equal to 2.

C. Serological tests
  1. Elevated RA factor more than 1:320
     OR
  2. Elevated anti nuclear antibody (ANA) more than 1:320
     OR
  3. Presence of anti SS-A/Ro and anti SS-B/La antibodies.

II. Secondary Sjögren's syndrome

Features of primary Sjögren's syndrome with Rheumatoid arthritis, polymyositis, scleroderma, biliary cirrhosis, etc.

Management of Sjögren's Syndrome

1. The goal of management in Sjögren's syndrome is to minimize the secondary effects of xerostomia on the oral cavity.
2. Salivary substitutes can be prescribed to the patients to keep their mouth wet.
3. Regular dental check ups and application of topical fluorides is beneficial to reduce the incidence of dental caries in these patients.
4. Nystatin, Clotrimazole and other anti fungal agents can be prescribed to treat candidiasis.
5. The patient must also be referred to an ophthalmologist for regular eye examination.

SALIVARY GLAND TUMORS

Pleomorphic Adenoma

(i) Pleomorphic adenoma is also known as mixed tumor because it is composed of different types of tissues such as fibrous, myxoid, chondroid or even osseous in addition to the salivary gland cells.

(ii) The parotid gland is the most common major salivary gland to be involved. Amongst the minor salivary glands, the palate is the most common site.

(iii) Lesions begin as slow growing, painless mass usually in elderly females (Fig. 13.10).

(iv) Lesions of minor salivary gland appear as well defined soft to firm swelling covered by a normal mucosa. When the tumor reaches large size, the mucosa may get ulcerated due to masticatory trauma.

(v) Investigations such as USG, CT scan and sialography can be performed to assess the size and extent of the lesion. An incisional biopsy or FNAC may be required to confirm the diagnosis (Fig. 13.11).

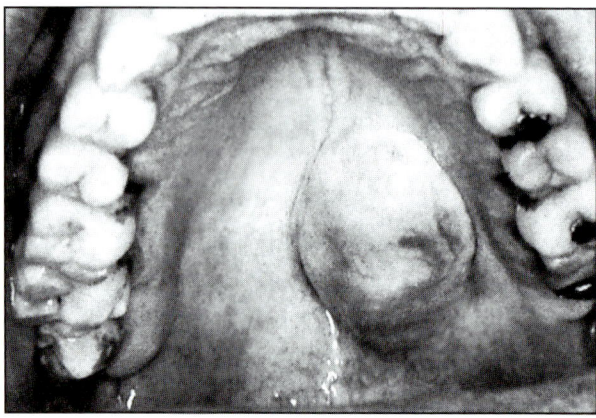

Fig. 13.10: A pleomorphic adenoma of the palate.

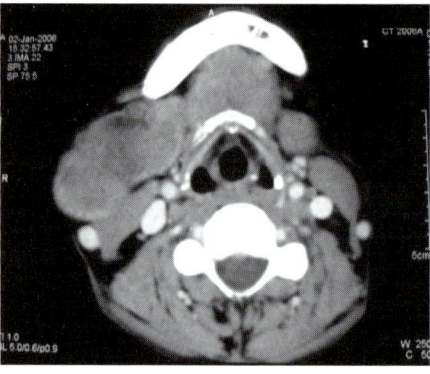

Fig. 13.11: CT scan showing a large pleomorphic adenoma of the submandibular gland.

(vi) Surgical removal of the gland/tumor is the treatment of choice. When the parotid gland is affected, superficial parotidectomy may be sufficient so that the facial nerve can be salvaged. Rarely pleomorphic adenoma may undergo malignant transformation and such lesions are known as carcinoma ex pleomorphic adenoma.

Papillary Cyst Adenoma Lymphomatosum (Warthin's Tumor)

(i) Warthin's tumor is a benign salivary gland tumor that almost exclusively affects the parotid gland. The tumor is believed to be arising from the intra parotid lymph nodes trapped within the gland.

(ii) The tumor affects elderly males more often and in characteristically bilateral arising from the tail of the parotid gland.

(iii) They are slow growing painless tumors, rarely attaining a large size.

(iv) Histologically, it shows a cystic lumen with cells giving in papillary projections into the lumen. The stroma shows abundance of lymphocytic infiltration.

(v) Appearance of hot spot in scintigraphy is an important diagnostic finding which occurs because of retention of the tracer within the tumor as the tumor cells do not communicate with the ductal lumen.

SUGGESTED READING AND REFERENCES

1. Oral Radiology. Principles and Interpretation: White and Pharoah, – 5th edition.
2. Essentials of Dental Radiography and Radiology. Eric Whaites, 3rd edition.
3. Principles and Practice of Oral Radiographic Interpretations – H.M.Worth.
4. Differential Diagnosis of Oral Lesions. Wood and Goaz.
5. Diseases of Salivary Glands. Rankow.
6. Oral and Maxillofacial Surgical Clinics of North America – Aug 1995.

Notes

CHAPTER 14

Temporomandibular Joint Disorders

The temporomandibular joint (TMJ) is a complex bilateral ginglymoarthrodial diarthrosis. The articulating surfaces are formed by the head of the condyle inferiorly and the glenoid fossa and articular eminence superiorly. The joint cavity is divided into a superior and inferior joint space by means of an intraarticular disc. The TM joints are anatomically two separate joints, but they function as a single joint, a feature that makes them unique. In other words, unlike any other joint in the body, at no point of time can only one of the TMJ function alone.

Classification of TM Joint Disorders

The various disorders that can affect the TMJ are classified as follows:

    I. *Developmental anomalies*
- (a) Condylar agenesis – unilateral/bilateral
- (b) Condylar hypoplasia
- (c) Condylar hyperplasia
- (d) Bifid condyle
- (e) Juvenile arthrosis
- (f) Coronoid hyperplasia

    II. *Degenerative joint disorders*
        Osteoarthritis – primary/secondary

    III *Inflammatory joint disorders*
        Rheumatoid arthritis

    IV. *Functional joint disorders*
- (a) Hypermobility
- (b) Ankylosis

V. *Traumatic disorders*
  (a) Subluxation and luxation
  (b) Fractures of the TMJ
VI. *Soft tissue abnormalities within the joint*
  (a) Internal disc derangement with reduction
  (b) Internal disc derangement without reduction
  (c) Disc perforation
VII. *Myofacial pain dysfunction syndrome (MPDS)*
VIII. *Neoplasms affecting the TMJ*

Condylar Hypoplasia

  (i) It is a developmental condition in which the condyles are small in size but have a normal morphology.
 (ii) The condition may be congenital or acquired. Causes of acquired hypoplasia include trauma to the TMJ during forceps delivery, irradiation to the joint in early age, infections of the joint, endocrine disturbances, etc.
(iii) The condition may be associated with other developmental anomalies like micrognathia, Treacher Collins syndrome.
 (iv) Asymmetry of the face is present and the chin deviates to the affected side on opening the mouth. Degenerative joint diseases set in as secondary complications.

Radiographic Features

  (a) The condyle is small, but normal in shape with thin, slender neck.
  (b) Neck of the condyle may be dorsally inclined.
  (c) Asymmetry of the jaw is present with dental crowding.
  (d) The ante gonial notch is deepened.
  (e) The sigmoid notch appears to have come in close proximity to the zygomatic arch.

D.D. This condition must be differentiated from other acquired anomalies such as degenerative joint disease and joint erosions caused due to rheumatoid arthritis.

Condylar Hyperplasia

  (i) It is a developmental condition characterized by large size of the condyle. Presence of over reactive cartilage at the growth sites in the condylar head may be responsible for such an overgrowth. Growth is usually self limiting and stops with completion of skeletal growth.

(ii) The patients present with a mandibular asymmetry, the chin deviated to the unaffected side. Malocclusions such as open bite on the affected side are common. The movements of the joint may be restricted owing to the large-sized condyle.

Radiographic Appearance

(a) Asymmetric enlargement of condyle is noted. A size difference of up to 3 mm between the two sides is considered to be a normal variation.

(b) The neck of the condyle is thickened and bent.

(c) However the normal cortical thickness and trabecular pattern can be seen (This features serves to distinguish them from a tumor.).

(d) A depression may be noted at the inferior border of the mandible where the affected side meets the normal side.

(e) Vertical depth of the ramus is increased.

(f) A Technetium 99m diphosphonate scan can be performed to study the persistent growth activity in the joint.

H.M.Worth has classified condylar hyperplasia into three types.

Type I : The condyle attempts to remodel and produces a normal shaped condyle which is large with a thickened neck.

Type II : No remodeling takes place. The enlarged condyle acquires an inverted 'L' shaped.

Type III : There is an exuberant response of the condyle to inflammation in the joint.

D.D.: The large-sized condyle must be differentiated from a neoplasm involving the joint.

Orthognathic surgery along with orthodontic therapy can be performed to correct the defect.

Bifid Condyle

A bifid condyle is a rare congenital anomaly where a deep notch or depression is seen on the head of the condyle in the frontal or sagittal plane. The condition can be unilateral or bilateral.

(i) Obstruction to the blood flow or longitudinal fractures of the condyle may be the cause of a bifid condyle.

(ii) Patients are asymptomatic and the condition is accidentally identified during routine radiographic examination on an OPG. A notch may be seen on the superior surface of the head of the condyle. Changes may also be present in the mandibular fossa to accommodate the altered shape of the condyle.

(iii) No treatment is indicated unless pain or dysfunction is present.

Juvenile Arthrosis (Boering's Arthrosis)

(i) This condition results from condylar growth disturbance that causes alteration in the shape of the condyle.

(ii) Patients are children and adolescents who may present with mandibular asymmetry along with signs and symptoms of dysfunction.

(iii) Radiographically, marked flattening of the condyle and apparent elongation of articular surface of the condyle give it a *toad stool appearance* (Fig. 14.1).

(iv) The neck of the condyle may be short or absent.

(v) The temporal component appears to be flattened.

(vi) The ramus is short with prominent antegonial notch.

Orthodontic treatment coupled with surgery can correct the asymmetry and prevent further destruction of the condyles.

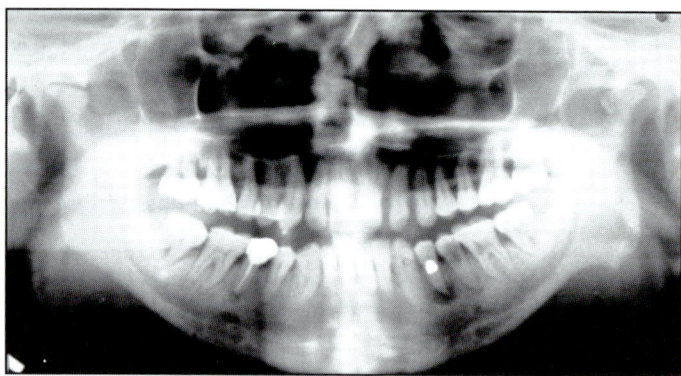

Fig. 14.1: OPG showing toadstool appearance of the condyles.

Coronoid Hyperplasia

(i) Hyperplasia of the coronoid process is an important differential diagnosis to be considered for progressive limitation of mouth opening.

(ii) The condition may be acquired or developmental.

(iii) The coronoid process extends more than 1 cm above the zygomatic arch and impinges on the medial surface of the arch, thus restricting the mouth opening.

(iv) Radiographically, the enlarged coronoid process acquires a *drumstick appearance* which may be seen on an OPG or Water's view.

D.D: Tumor involving the coronoid process must be differentiated from hyperplasia.

OSTEOARTHRITIS

Articular remodeling is a biological process which allows the morphology of the joints to change in response to stress. If the biomechanical stress exceeds the remodeling capacity of the joint, degenerative changes set in. Osteoarthritis is thus primarily a non-inflammatory process involving the deterioration of the articular soft tissues and remodeling of the underlying bone. The earliest change is freying of the articular surfaces of both the temporal and condylar bones. Eventually, the articular surfaces become completely denuded and the eburnated bone comes in direct contact with the meniscus. If this process continues, then excessive erosion of the bone occurs with sclerosis of the underlying bone, sub condylar cysts and peripheral osteophyte formation. Such a change may also be as a response to chronic microtrauma or pressure caused due to age or parafunctional habits such as bruxism and clenching.

Clinical Features

(i) Pain over the joint is a frequent complaint of the patient.

(ii) The patient may complain of a feeling of stiffness after a period of inactivity.

(iii) Mouth opening may be restricted accompanied by tenderness and crepitus.

(iv) The jaw may deviate to the affected side on opening the mouth.

Radiographic Features

(i) In very early stages, bone changes may not be apparent on the radiograph.

(ii) Narrowing of the joint space may be noticed on the radiograph.

(iii) Flattening of the articulating surfaces and sub chondral sclerosis may be evident which indicate previous remodeling (Fig. 14.2).

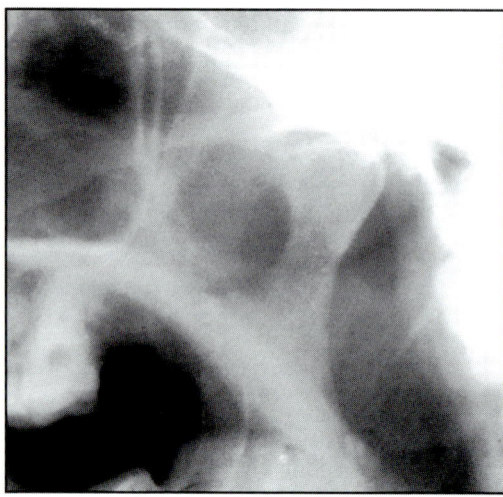

Fig. 14.2: Radiograph showing flattening and breaking of the condyle due to arthritis.

(iv) Osteophyte formation and lipping of the bone appears which are best visualized on the CT scan.

(v) Over a period of time, these osteophytes may get detached from the bone and lie freely in the joint space. They are referred to as joint mice.

(vi) Areas of degeneration containing granulation tissue are formed within the head of the condyle that appear as radiolucencies known as Ely's cyst.

(vii) Sometimes, the temporal component may also show erosions along the posterior slope of the articular eminence.

Treatment of Osteoarthritis

1. The presence of any parafunctional habits must be identified and corrected. Soft acrylic splints worn at night can help to reduce the impact of such potentially detrimental habit on the joint.

2. Symptomatic relief from pain can be sought by prescribing analgesics such as Ibuprofen (400 mg tds, for 5–10 days), Piroxicam.

3. Soft diet, restricted mouth opening and hot fomentations over the joint are also effective palliative measures in relieving joint pain and stiffness.

4. Surgery to remove the osteophyte or arthroplasty can be performed if the condition is very severe and does not respond to conventional therapy.

RHEUMATOID ARTHRITIS

(i) Rheumatoid arthritis is a disease that is characterized by inflammation of the synovial lining of the joint which leads to synovial granulomatous tissue called *pannus* growing into the articular surfaces of the joint. Further release of enzymes results in destruction of bone and the joint.

(ii) It is a disease that affects multiple joints in the body, usually beginning with the interphalangeal and wrist joints.

(iii) TMJ involvement may be unilateral or bilateral affecting predominantly the females.

(iv) Patients have a long series of exacerbations and remissions. They complain of pain and swelling in the joint.

(v) Movements are painful and restricted especially early in the morning. Symptoms gradually improve during the day with continued movements in contrast to patients with osteoarthritis in whom the pain and symptoms worsens with movements.

(vi) Severe joint involvement can cause erosion of the condyle resulting in anterior open bite.

Radiographic Features

(i) Osteopenia and reduced density of the bone are early radiographic changes seen in rheumatoid arthritis.

(ii) Erosions of the head of condyle and articular eminence can be seen that results in anterosuperior positioning of the condyle and open bite.

(iii) Typically the anterior and posterior surfaces of the condyles undergo erosion and the condyle acquires a *sharpened pencil* appearance.

(iv) In extremely severe cases, the condyle may be completely lost and replaced by a concavity.

Treatment of Rheumatoid Arthritis

1. Pain relief can be obtained with anti-inflammatory drugs.

2. Soft diet, hot fomentation and physiotherapy are valuable adjuvants in the management of pain and restoration of function.

3. Intraarticular injections of steroids and gold salt therapy can be considered in advanced cases.

4. When the joint has been completely destroyed by the disease, replacement with a suitable prosthesis can be considered.

ANKYLOSIS

(i) It is an extremely debilitating condition characterized by inability to open the mouth that severely affects oral function. Difficulty in maintaining oral hygiene also predisposes to dental caries and periodontal diseases.

(ii) Ankylosis may be of the following types:
True/False ankylosis
Fibrous/Bony ankylosis

Etiology of Ankylosis

The following causes have been proposed for the occurrence of ankylosis.

(a) Trauma during birth such as due to forceps delivery.

(b) Infection of the middle ear spreading to the TMJ.

(c) Untreated TMJ fractures.

(d) Prolonged immobilization of jaws in children.

Clinical Features

(i) Mouth opening is reduced and the mandible appears to be retruded. This gives rise to a *bird face appearance* (Fig. 14.3).

(ii) The movements on the affected side are decreased and may not be palpable.

(iii) The chin deviates to the affected side on attempting to open the mouth. The

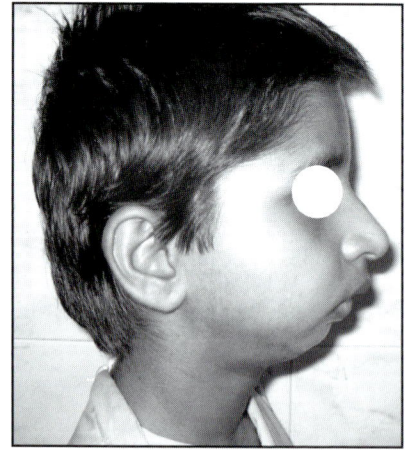

Fig. 14.3: Bird face appearance of the face due to ankylosis of the TMJ.

muscles of the neck such as the sternocleidomastoid and trapezius become prominent when the patient tries to open his mouth forcefully.

(iv) Severe malocclusion is present with the teeth arranged horizontally in the ramus.

Radiographic Features

(i) The joint space may be completely or partially missing and replaced by a chunk of irregular bone.

(ii) The condylar outline is not traceable on the radiographs.

(iii) The ante gonial notches are prominent because of lack of action of lateral pterygoid muscle or hyperfunction of closing muscles and supra hyoid muscles. The ramus is short.

(iv) There is compensatory coronoid hyperplasia which can be seen on an OPG..

(v) Severe crowding of the teeth may be present. The teeth are placed horizontally in the ramus, as the condylar growth center is not active, the teeth continue to remain in the vertical ramus.

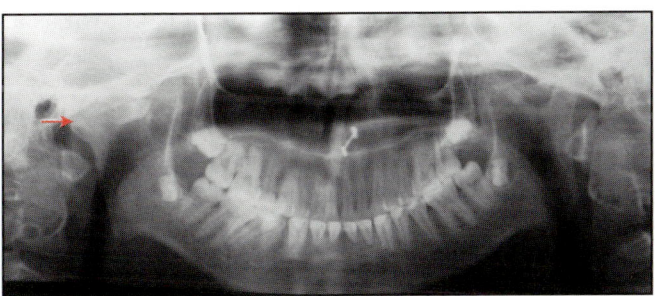

Fig. 14.4: OPG showing the characteristic radiographic features of TMJ ankylosis (arrow).

Treatment of Ankylosis

Surgical correction with gap arthroplasty and other techniques are the treatment of choice to correct the deformity and restore the function.

INTERNAL DISC DERANGEMENT

Farrar and McCarthy have defined disc displacement as anterior displacement of the disk associated with postero-superior positioning of the condyle in the closed mouth position.

Etiology

(i) Chronic low grade microtrauma to the joint due to habits, such as bruxism and clenching is known to be the cause of disc displacement. Such a constant action results in laxity of the joint.

(ii) Indirect trauma to the joints due to sudden cervical flexion as during a whiplash injury can also result into displacement of the disc.

(iii) Some authors postulate that the disc is nothing but an extended tendon of the upper head of lateral pterygoid muscle. Thus abnormal functioning of lateral pterygoid muscle is also considered to be one of the etiological factors in disc displacement.

Normal Disc Condyle Relationship

In a normal joint, the disc lies above the head of the condyle, inserted anteriorly into the superior head of lateral pterygoid and posteriorly to the posterior attachment and retrodiscal tissues which are made of elastic cartilage. As the condyle translates anteriorly during mouth opening, the disc gets stretched and comes to lie between the head of the condyle and the articular eminence. During closure of the mouth, the condyles move backwards and the disc recoils to its normal position. The normal appearance of the biconcave disc as seen on an MRI scan is known as a *bow-tie appearance*.

Anterior Disc Displacement with Reduction

In this condition, during the normal rest position, the disc lies displaced with the posterior band lying anteriorly. However when the mouth is opened, it snaps back to its normal location between the head of condyle and the articular eminence producing a *click*. Once again when the mouth is closed, the disc returns to its dislocated position.

Anterior Disc Displacement Without Reduction

In this condition, the disc remains in a displaced position anteriorly in the closed mouth position. Even when the mouth is opened, it does not reduce to its normal position, but gets folded and compressed locking itself creating a *gum ball effect* (Fig. 14.5).

Clinical Features

(i) Disc displacements do not always produce clinical symptoms.

(ii) Patients may have reduced movements of the jaw and opening the mouth may be at times very painful.

(iii) Deviation of the jaw to the affected side may be observed on opening the mouth.

(iv) A click sound can be heard while the patient opens his mouth indication the movement of the disc. A similar but a softer click is heard as the patient closes his mouth indicating that the disc has once again attained its displaced position.

(v) Clicking sound may be absent in non reducing discs instead a crepitus which is a grating or sound may be heard on opening and closing the mouth.

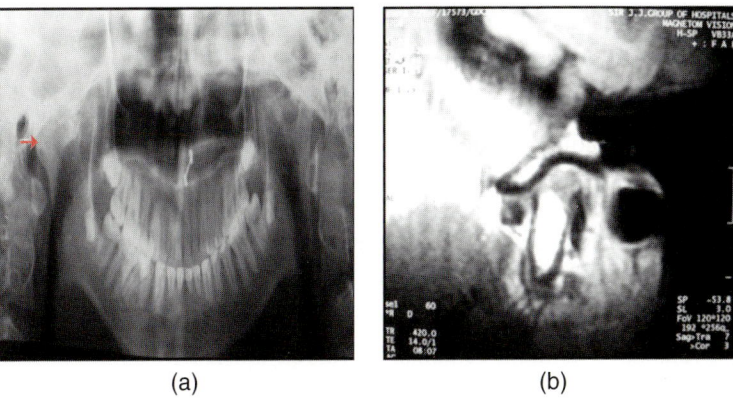

(a)   (b)

Figs 14.5a and b: (a) MRI scan showing disc in the closed mouth position (b) MRI scan showing non-reducing disc in the open mouth position.

Radiographic Features

(a) Conventional radiography cannot show the location of the disc. MRI scans are the best to study disc displacements.

(b) Arthrography can be performed in which a radiopaque dye is injected into the upper and lower joint spaces and radiographs are made which demonstrate the disc position.

Treatment of Disc Displacements

Patients with disc displacements can be treated by providing anterior repositioning splints. Conservative therapy for pain relief with analgesics, physiotherapy should be considered.

MYOFACIAL PAIN DYSFUNCTION SYNDROME (MPDS)

MPDS or Costen's syndrome is a disease entity that results from spasm of the muscles supporting the jaws due to multiple causes most important being overclosure or overextension of the muscles.

Etiology

The various factors that have been associated in the cause of MPDS are as follows:

(i) Parafunctional habits, e.g. nocturnal bruxing, tooth clenching, lip or cheek biting.

(ii) Emotional distress.

(iii) Acute trauma from blows or impacts.

(iv) Trauma from hyperextension, e.g. dental procedures, oral intubation for general anesthesia, yawning, hyperextension associated with cervical trauma.

(v) Instability of maxillomandibular relationships.

(vi) Laxity of the joint.

(vii) Comorbidity of other rheumatic or musculoskeletal disorders.

(viii) Poor general health and an unhealthy lifestyle.

Pathophysiology of MPDS (Laskin's theory)

The pathophysiology of MPDS emphasizes mainly on the muscular tension caused by oral habits and dental irritants. The following flow chart gives a lucid explanation to the mechanism involved in MPDS.

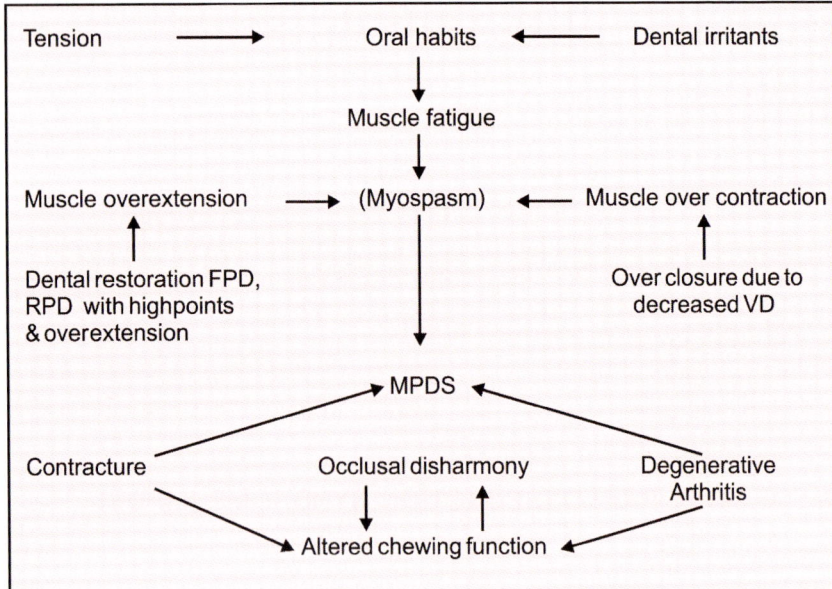

Clinical Features

1. Patients complain of unilateral, dull pain in the ear or preauricular region.
2. Pain is worse on awakening in the morning.
3. Tenderness of muscle of mastication is present.
4. Mouth opening is limited and painful. The jaw deviates to affected side on opening the mouth.

Laskin's four cardinal signs of MPDS:

(a) Unilateral pain: There must be a dull ache in the preauricular region. Pain is worse on waking up.
(b) Muscle tenderness must be present on palpation.
(c) Clicking/popping noise must be heard in the TMJ.
(d) Mouth opening must be restricted.

Negative Features

(a) Absence of radiographic findings.
(b) Lack of tenderness in the TMJ on palpation from the external auditory meatus.

Trigger Points

These are localized deep tenderness in areas of taut band of skeletal muscle, tendon or ligament that has the tendency to cause referred pain in a definite anatomic distribution when stimulated. Presence of such trigger points are characteristic feature of MPDS. The area perceived by the irritable trigger point is called the zone of reference. In MPDS, pain is elicited by applying digital pressure on the trigger point whereas in trigeminal neuralgia, even a light touch or breeze is sufficient to stimulate the trigger zone and precipitate an attack of pain.

Jump Sign

It is the withdrawal of head, wrinkling of head or verbal response given by the patient on palpating the trigger points.

Tanaka's recommendations for palpation of muscles.

(i) Muscle must be evaluated in its entire length including its origin and insertion.
(ii) The muscles must be evaluated in rest and contracted position.
(iii) The muscles must be examined bilaterally to compare the difference.

(iv) The muscles must be palpated horizontally and vertically to the attachments.

While palpating the muscles, begin palpating with light pressures before proceeding to 3–4 pounds. Muscle palpation may be performed by two methods, i.e.

Flat palpation: When muscle can be palpated over the bone, e.g. masseter.

Pincer palpation: When the belly of the muscle can be held between the fingers, e.g. sternocleidomastoid.

Treatment Consideration

Multiple therapeutic approach is preferred in the management of MPDS beginning with patient education and counseling.

I. Pharmacotherapy

1. NSAIDs are the drug of choice for immediate pain relief. Ibuprofen 400 mg tds or Nimesulide 100 mg BD are good choices of analgesics.

2. Diclofenac gel in pluronic lecithin organogel can be rubbed over the skin followed by hot fomentation which gives relief from pain and improves mouth opening.

3. Muscle relaxants such as Chloroxazone 250 mg tid, Carisoprodol 350 mg tid (tab Soma) are valuable in reducing muscle spasm.

4. Amitriptyline which is a tricyclic antidepressant can be given in the doses of 10 or 25 mg at bed time to reduce patient anxiety and provide a good refreshing sleep.

II. Intraoral Appliance Therapy

Hard and soft splints can be fabricated that help to unload TMJ and establish a harmonious relation between TMJ and muscles.

III. Trigger Point Therapy

The spray and stretch technique provides stimulation of cutaneous afferent nerves and produces trigger point inhibition causing pain relief. Fluromethane spray is an effective choice for the same.

Alternatively injection of local anesthesia 0.5% procaine, bupivacaine into the trigger points reduces pain. However chances of myotoxicity and other reactions should be considered before initiating the therapy.

IV. Relaxation Therapy

This mode of therapy decreases sympathetic activity and arousal. Brief methods such as deep breathing and deep methods such as meditation, progressive muscle relaxation can be performed under the supervision of a trained master to provide muscle relaxation.

V. Physiotherapy

Various types of treatments like moist heat, ultrasound and short wave diathermy help immensely in reducing pain and dysfunction. They act by increasing the vascularity of the muscle, resolution of inflammation and fibrosis and increasing the flexibility of connective tissue. Isokinetic exercises of the jaws also provide a similar effect to the muscles.

Other methods such as massage, accupressure, homeopathic and herbal medicines, botulinum toxin are also used widely in the treatment of MPDS.

SUGGESTED READING AND REFERENCES

1. Oral Radiology. Principles and Interpretation: White and Pharoah 5th edition.
2. Essentials of Dental Radiography and Radiology. Eric Whaites, 3rd edition.
3. Principles and Practice of Oral Radiographic Interpretations— H.M.Worth.
4. Common Diseases of TMJ. Ogus and Toller.
5. Panoramic Radiology. Langland.
6. TMJ Disorders and Orofacial Pain. DCNA Jan 2007.
7. TMJ Imaging. Christiansen.

Notes

15

Diseases of Maxillary Sinus

The maxillary sinuses are a pair of air filled cavities located within the body of the maxilla. They communicate with the nasal cavity through an ostium which drains into the middle meatus. The sinuses are lined by pseudostratified ciliated columnar epithelium. Though the function of these sinuses in not clear, it is proposed that they serve to humidify and warm the inhaled air and add resonance to the voice in addition to lightening the skull.

Classification of Diseases of Maxillary Sinus

   I. *Inflammatory disease (Sinusitis)*
- (a) Acute
- (b) Chronic

  II. *Traumatic lesions*
- (a) Concussion or laceration of the sinus mucosa.
- (b) Blow out fractures of the orbit involving the sinus.
- (c) Isolated fractures of the sinus.
- (d) Complex fractures associated with middle third injuries.
- (e) Oro-antral fistula.

 III. *Cystic lesions*
- (a) Intrinsic cyst: mucous retention cyst, benign mucosal cyst, surgical ciliated cyst.
- (b) Extrinsic cysts: Dentigerous cyst, Radicular cyst, OKC, etc.

 IV. *Neoplastic diseases*
- (a) Benign tumors
  - Papilloma
  - Osteoma
  - Ameloblastoma

- AOT
- Complex odontoma
- Ossifying fibroma
  (b) Malignant tumors
    - Squamous cell carcinoma
    - Adenocarcinomas
  V. *Fibrous dysplasia*

Examination of the Patient with Maxillary Sinus Disease

In addition to the routine history taking and examination, the following specific factors must be considered while examining a patient with maxillary sinus disease.

1. The patient must be examined for any asymmetry, ecchymosis, deformity and erythema of the skin over the sinus. These may be signs of traumatic injury involving the sinus.
2. Presence of epistaxis and epiphora are signs of malignant tumor or space occupying lesion within the sinus.
3. Paresthesia of the infraorbital nerve may be present which should alert the clinician of a fracture involving the sinus wall or a malignant tumor.
4. Tenderness of teeth in the absence of any dental pathology may be a feature of sinusitis. Such teeth are referred to as *Stomp positive*, i.e. they are painful when the patient jumps or walks fast.
5. Trismus may be caused due to tumors of the maxillary sinus destroying the posterior wall of the sinus and invading the pterygoid muscles or locking of the coronoid process.
6. Eye movements must be noted carefully. Visual disturbance is associated with blow out fractures and also malignant tumors involving the orbit.
7. Cervical lymph nodes must be examined in all the cases as they are enlarged in infections and malignant tumors of the sinus.

Radiological Evaluation of a Patient with Maxillary Sinus Disease

The following investigations may be performed for a case of suspected maxillary sinus disease.

1. Radiographs

Radiographic survey is the preliminary choice of investigation of sinus disease. IOPA views can be made to study the floor of sinus, diagnose and locate oro-antral fistula and displaced root pieces. For large lesions, lateral occlusal views can be made to visualize the sinus and its floor.

Amongst the extraoral views, OPG and Water's view are the most important views to study the sinuses. As a rule cystic lesions are better visualized on OPG while haziness of the sinus due to sinusitis can be studied more clearly on the Water's view. The posterior wall of the sinus cannot be seen on the Water's view and an SMV view is required to demonstrate this.

The normal sinus contains air and hence appears radiolucent. Any pathology or change within the sinus encroaches the air space and hence appears a relatively radiopaque. The radiographic appearances of sinus disease is thus not specific owing to the fact that transudates, exudates, blood will all produce a similar shadow on the radiograph.

2. CT Scans

CT scans are excellent choice to study various pathologies involving the sinus including sinusitis, cysts, tumors, fractures, etc. Coronal and axial sections must be obtained to study the entire extent of the lesions. CT scans are mandatory in cases of fractures and malignant tumors involving the sinus.

3. MRI Scans

MRI scans produce an excellent soft tissue contrast and valuable in studying cyst and tumors involving the sinus. Mucosal thickening of the sinus wall and accumulation of fluid within the sinus can be studied with MRI scans.

4. Radionuclide Scanning

Scans obtained after injection of a radioisotope such as ^{99m}Tc demonstrate the physiological changes taking place within the sinus. Scintigraphic studies are useful in the diagnosis of malignant tumors of the sinus to study the complete extent of the tumor.

Maxillary Sinusitis

(i) Sinusitis can be due to bacterial or allergic cause. *Haemophilus influenzae*, *Streptococcus pneumoniae* are the common causative organisms of maxillary sinusitis. A rare cause can be due to fungal infection such as aspergillosis which is usually seen in immunocompromised patients.

(ii) Conditions such as deviated nasal septum (DNS) predispose to sinusitis. Spread of infection from the oral cavity from an infected root apex or displaced root piece can also lead to sinusitis.

(iii) Nasal congestion or obstructions accompanied with head ache and secretion from the nose are considered as the triad of sinusitis.

Radiographic Features

(a) The thickening of the mucosa and accumulation of secretion during sinusitis reduces the air content of the sinus and causes the sinus to appear increasingly radiopaque. The thickened mucosa appears nearly parallel to the walls of the sinus. It may be of uniform thickness or polypoid.

(b) In chronic sinusitis, opacification of sinus takes place which may be accompanied by sclerosis of the bony walls.

(c) The presence of fluid within the sinus can be ascertained if the line of demarcation between the opacity and the sinus is straight and horizontal. Fluid level indicates pus or blood in the sinus. The radiograph must be made in a standing position to confirm this feature.

Treatment of Sinusitis

1. In early stages, antibiotic therapy with steam inhalation is a good method of treating sinusitis. Amoxycillin and cephalosporin provide good coverage against the organisms involved in acute maxillary sinusitis.

2. In severe cases, surgical drainage may have to be established to relieve the patient.

3. Chronic maxillary sinusitis cases may require a Caldwell Luc operation to curette the sinus contents or correction of DNS to avoid recurrence.

Empyema

Sometimes the ostium of the sinus gets blocked by thickened mucosa or other pathologic conditions. In such cases the pus accumulates inside the sinus. Such an accumulation of pus within a cavity is known as empyema. Radiographically, the sinus appears to be completely opacified. Such opacity must be differentiated from simple mucosal thickening. Accumulation of pus inside the sinus may lead to osteomyelitis.

Mucous Retention Cyst of the Antrum

This is a common sequelae of an inflamed or hyperplastic lining of the maxillary sinus. Retention cysts are formed when the duct of a seromucinous gland is blocked or damaged due to inflammatory reaction. The lesion is usually unilateral, asymptomatic and accidentally discovered during a routine radiographic survey.

Radiographic Features

The cyst appears as a dome-shaped radiopacity attached to the floor or lateral wall of the sinus. An OPG is a clear view to identify such cyst. If the cyst is large, it may fill up the entire maxillary sinus and appear as uniform cloudiness. Sometimes a large cyst may protrude through the ostium into the sinus.

The differential diagnosis for such cystic lesions inside the sinus includes odontogenic cysts. The presence of a hyperostotic border around the cyst that appears as a white line serves to identify odontogenic cysts which are extrinsic in origin. Antral polyps must also be differentiated where mucosal thickening of the entire antral lining is present.

Contusions of the Sinus

A blow on the face may transmit the force through the bone of the anterior wall of the sinus causing a tear in the mucosal lining. The anterolateral wall may suffer a greenstick fracture but sometimes since this bone is relatively elastic; it gives rise to laceration of the sinus mucosa and bleeding within the sinus.

Radiographic Features

Contusions of the maxillary sinus appear as haziness of the sinus due to bleeding. Fluid level can be demonstrated on a radiograph made in a standing position.

Blow Out Fractures

When the globe of the eye sustains a blunt injury due to an object larger than its size, the kinetic energy is converted into hydraulic energy and the orbital contents break the floor and the medial wall. Thus it causes herniation of the orbital contents into the sinus.

Clinical features of blow out fractures include peri-orbital edema, sub conjunctival ecchymosis, hooding of eye/enophthalmus and diplopia.

Radiographic Signs Include

   (i) Soft tissue swelling over the orbital rim.

  (ii) Trap door sign or bright light sign on the CT.

 (iii) Polypoid density in the roof of the sinus.

 (iv) Teardrop herniation of the orbital contents into the sinus.

  (v) If the distance between infraorbital margin and floor of orbit appears more than 2 mm on PA Water's view it is suggestive of fracture of the floor of orbit.

Oro-antral Fistula/Communication

Oro-antral fistula (OAF) is an unnatural communication between the oral cavity and the maxillary sinus. The term fistula is used to denote communication between the oral cavity and the antrum which is chronic and lined by the epithelium. The most important cause for the formation of an OAF is iatrogenic perforation of the floor of sinus during extraction of an upper molar with the root piece displaced into the sinus. Other causes include, traumatic injuries to the maxilla such as gunshot injuries, infections such as syphilis causing perforation of the palate.

Clinical Features

   (i) Sudden disappearance of a root piece during extraction into the socket is a sign of an oro-antral communication.

  (ii) Bubbling of the blood clot when the patient blows his nose also suggests a newly formed fistula.

 (iii) Regurgitation of fluids, nasal twang in the voice and features of chronic sinusitis may be seen in long-standing cases.

 (iv) A mouth mirror held near the orifice turns moist when the patient blows with his nostrils closed. Similarly a wisp of cotton will flutter when it is held near the perforation when the patient blows his nose.

Radiographic Feature

  (a) Discontinuity of the floor of sinus can be seen on an IOPA view or lateral occlusal view.

  (b) The displaced root piece may be present inside the sinus and appears as a radiopaque mass with a radiolucent root canal inside it.

  (c) In chronic cases, there may be generalized haziness of the sinus due to chronic inflammation.

D.D.: Must include a foreign body in the sinus, antrolith, normal bony projections within the sinus, etc.

Treatment of OAF

An OAF must be closed as soon as it is identified. The root piece may be retrieved through the socket or by a Caldwell Luc surgery. The fistula can be closed by various surgical procedures like buccal advancement flap, palatal advancement flap or a combination flap can be performed to close the fistula.

Antrolith

An antrolith is a calcified mass within the sinus. Antroliths form around endogenous foci such as inspissated pus, mucous plug, blood clot, etc. or around exogenous foci such as a foreign body, a piece of paper.

Antroliths are often asymptomatic but occasional large stones may perforate the medial wall of the sinus and protrude into the nasal cavity. Radiographically, they appear as round, oval or irregular shaped calcified masses within the sinus. It may also show alternate radiolucent and radiopaque lamellae.

EXTRINSIC CYSTS

Extrinsic cysts are those that arise outside the sinus and invade the sinus. The common extrinsic cysts include radicular cysts, dentigerous cysts, fissural cysts such as globulomaxillary cysts. They may be odontogenic or non odontogenic in origin.

Radicular cysts appear as periapical radiolucency in relation to the apex of a non-vital tooth. They have a corticated border that separates them from the sinus.

Dentigerous cysts are associated with the crown of an unerupted tooth. They appear as peri coronal radiolucency attached to the neck of the tooth. The associated impacted tooth may be pushed deep into the sinus at times reaching the floor of the orbit or the posterior wall of the sinus. A corticated wall separates the cyst from the sinus. CT scans must be obtained to confirm the location of the tooth inside the sinus.

Globulomaxillary cyst is a fissural cyst that arises from the epithelial remnants at the site of fusion of the maxilla and pre maxilla. It appears on the radiograph as pear shaper radiolucency between the canine and lateral incisor. A large expanding cyst may cause displacement of the walls of nasal cavity. The inverted 'Y' line of Ennis may be obliterated when such large cysts encroach the sinus.

BENIGN TUMORS

Benign tumors such as papilloma and osteoma arise within the sinus. Epithelial papilloma is a soft tissue mass arising from the lining of the walls of the sinus. Radiographically it appears haziness within the sinus.

Osteomas are the most common mesenchymal tumors of the PNS. It is a slowly growing expansile lesion causing nasal obstruction. The frontal sinus is the most common sinus to be affected. On the radiographs, osteomas appear as lobulated sharply defined, rounded homogeneous mass of much greater opacity.

Extrinsic tumors involving the sinus include ameloblastoma, AOT.

The most common extrinsic tumor affecting the sinus is ameloblastoma. It is an aggressive tumor when it occurs in the maxilla and grows rapidly causing loosening of the teeth and nasal obstruction. It also causes painless deformity of the middle third of the face. Radiographically it appears as unilocular or multilocular radiolucency involving the sinus. The complete extension of ameloblastoma can be studied on a CT scan.

AOT is a benign odontogenic tumor chiefly affecting the anterior part of the maxilla. It may extend posteriorly to involve the sinus. The lesion present as an expansile radiolucent mass having an impacted tooth or areas of calcification with a *Milky Way appearance* of the lumen.

SQUAMOUS CELL CARCINOMA OF THE SINUS

It accounts to about 3% of malignant tumors affecting the sinus. The clinical features depend upon the walls of the sinus that are affected.

 (i) When the medial wall is affected, it causes nasal symptoms such as nasal obstruction, discharge, epistaxis and pain.

 (ii) When the floor is affected, it causes numbness of the teeth, unusual mobility of the teeth and swelling of the palate.

 (iii) When the lateral wall is affected, it causes swelling on the face and vestibule along with pain and hyperesthesia of the maxillary teeth.

 (iv) When the roof of the sinus is affected, eye symptoms such as diplopia, proptosis, pain in the cheeks and upper teeth are the presenting feature and sometimes sudden loss of vision may take place.

(v) When the tumor spreads posteriorly, the pterygoid muscles are affected and this along with locking of the coronoid process causes trismus and obstruction to the eustachian tube.

Radiographically, the tumor appears as haziness of the sinus. The affected walls of the sinus are destroyed and appear discontinuous (Fig. 15.1). CT scan, MRI and scintigraphy are important modalities in diagnosing this malignant tumor. Treatment involves surgical removal of the maxilla followed by radiotherapy and rehabilitation with a suitable prosthesis.

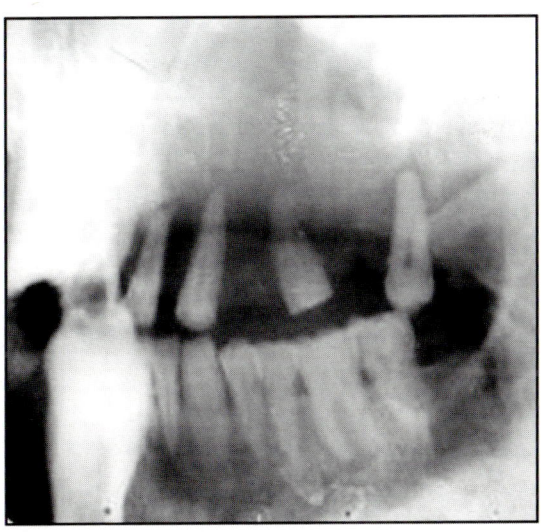

Fig. 15.1: Radiograph showing a malignant tumor in the maxilla causing destruction of its floor.

FIBROUS DYSPLASIA OF BONE

It is a benign fibro-osseous lesion that frequently affects the maxillary sinus. It is believed to be a hamartoma that has limited growth potential. Fibrous dysplasias commonly affect young individuals and presents as expansile dense radiopaque mass filling the sinus (Fig. 15.2). It may have a characteristic ground glass, stippled or a granular appearance. It is treated by surgical shaving of the excess bone which is best performed after the growth has stopped to avoid recurrence.

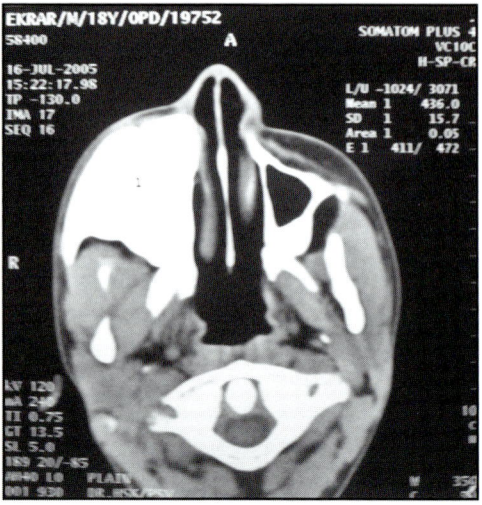

Fig. 15.2: CT scan showing fibrous dysplasia involving the right maxillary sinus.

SUGGESTED READING AND REFERENCES

1. Oral Radiology. Principles and Interpretation: White and Pharoah, 5th edition.
2. Essentials of Dental Radiography and Radiology. Eric Whaites, 3rd edition.
3. Principles and Practice of Oral Radiographic Interpretations— H.M.Worth.
4. The Maxillary Sinus and its Dental Implications. David Mc gowen
5. Panoramic Radiology. Langland.

CHAPTER 16

Fibro-osseous Lesions of the Jaws

Fibro-osseous lesions are a group of conditions with a common feature where there is replacement of bone by a tissue composed of collagen fibres and fibroblast that contain varying amounts of mineralized tissue. The term fibro-osseous is thus descriptive and diagnostically non specific.

Classification of Fibro-osseous Lesions

I. Fibrous dysplasia
   a. Monostotic
   b. Polyostotic

II. Fibro-osseous cemental lesions presumably arising from the PDL
   a. PCD
   b. Local cemental lesions
   c. FOD
   d. Ossifying fibroma/cementifying fibroma

III. Fibro-osseous lesions of uncertain/debatable relation to those arising from the PDL
   a. Cemento/osteoblastoma, osteoid osteoma
   b. Juvenile ossifying fibroma

Periapical Cemental Dysplasia

(i) It is also known as periapical osteofibrosis or cementoma. It is a condition in which the bone at the apex is replaced by fibrous tissue which then undergoes peripheral ossification initially and later on gets completely replaced by bone.

(ii) The mandibular anterior teeth in black females are most frequently affected.

(iii) These teeth are vital teeth and there is no H/O pain/sensitivity.

(iv) Large lesions can cause expansion of bone.

Radiographic Features

(a) In the early stages, it appears as well/ill-defined radiolucency less than 1 cm.

(b) The epicenter of the lesion lies over the root apex and the lesions are often multiple and bilateral.

(c) In the matured stage the lesions may be seen as mixed radiopaque and radiolucent areas in the apical region of the teeth.

(d) The radiopacity within the lesion is devoid of trabeculae.

(e) Multiple radiopaque masses may coalesce to form a single large mass surrounded by a radiolucent line.

(f) Radiopaque cemental masses may be left behind in the edentulous jaw after the affected ones have been extracted.

D.D.:

1. Periapical rarefying osteitis: The affected teeth are non vital.

2. Cementoblastoma: The lesion is solitary, attached to the root.

3. Odontoma: They usually occur coronal to the tooth, tooth like densities with a well-defined capsule can be seen radiographically.

FIBROUS DYSPLASIA

The term Fibrous dysplasia was given by Lichtenstein in 1938. It is also known as Fibrocystic disease, Osteitis fibrosa localisata, Focal osteitis fibrosa or Fibro-osteodystrophy.

Etiology

It was considered that fibrous dysplasia is a non specific developmental disturbance of the bone. Some investigators suggest that it is a hamartoma and has a limited growth potential. Recent studies have identified that mutation of GNAS 1 gene (Guanine nucleotide binding protein α stimulating activity polypeptide 1 gene) is responsible for the growth disturbance in the bone that results in fibrous dysplasia. The severity and manifestation of this disease depend on the time of mutation of the GNAS gene, e.g. mutation during the early embryonic stage affects the osteoblast, melanocytes, endocrine cells and results in Albright's syndrome. Mutation during the later stages before birth affects a progeny of cells thus causing multiple bone involvement and polyostotic form of disease. Mutations during the post-natal life result in a localized defect and thus manifests as monostotic form of fibrous dysplasia.

Types of Fibrous Dysplasias (FD)

I. Monostotic: involving only one bone.

II. Craniofacial type: involving many facial bones including the base of the skull.

III. Polyostotic: involving multiple bones in the body.

IV. Jaffe's syndrome: Fibrous dysplasia with café-au-lait spots.

Albright's syndrome: Fibrous dysplasia with café-au-lait spots and endocrine abnormality such as sexual precocity, gynaecomastia, premature spermatogenesis, pituitary adenoma, hyperparathyroidism.

CAFE-AU-LAIT SPOTS

These are unilateral tan macules that occur on the thighs, trunk, genital, oral cavity. They are so called because of their color which looks like *coffee with milk*. Café-au-lait spots are not specific findings in fibrous dysplasia but may also be seen in neurofibromatosis, Addison's disease and Albright's syndrome. Café-au-lait spots in Albright's syndrome have an irregular outline and resemble the *coast of Maine*, while those in neurofibromatosis have a smooth outline and resemble the *coast of California*.

Clinical Features

(i) Lesions begin growing in the early childhood; females are more frequently affected than males. The lesions may be activated during pregnancy or with the use of oral contraceptives.

(ii) It presents as a painless slow growing swelling (Fig. 16.1).

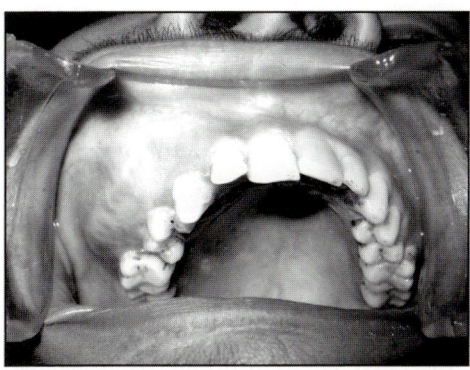

Fig. 16.1: Fibrous dysplasia causing expansion of the maxilla.

   (iii) The lesion in unilateral and the posterior part of maxilla is more frequently affected than the mandible.

   (iv) The craniofacial type is characterized by involvement of maxilla, zygoma, sphenoid and occiput.

Radiographic Features

   (a) Fibrous dysplasia typically causes enlargement of bone from within causing ribbon like thinning of cortex.

   (b) The early lesions appear as cyst-like radiolucency in the jaws.

   (c) The lamina dura of the teeth in the affected part of the bone become indistinct.

   (d) The radiopacity is poorly demarcated and blends imperceptibly.

   (e) The vertical depth of mandible is increased. In the maxilla, lesions encroach the sinus from the lateral wall (Fig. 16.4).

   (f) Superior displacement of the canal is another typical finding in fibrous dysplasia.

   (g) The internal trabecular pattern is altered and may give rise to various appearances such as *orange peel (Fig.16.3), thumb print or a ground glass (Fig. 16.2).*

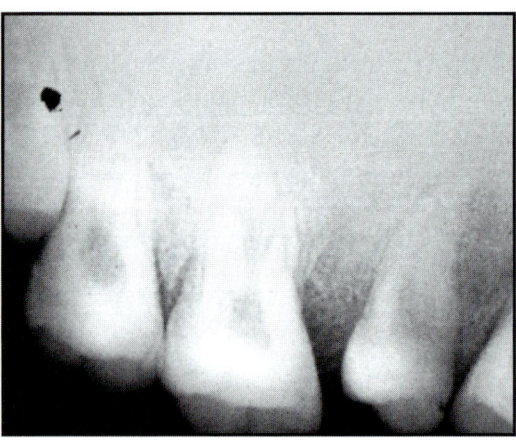

Fig. 16.2: IOPA radiograph showing ground glass appearance of fibrous dysplasia.

D.D.

   1. Dental cyst: Early stages of fibrous dysplasia may resemble a cyst which has a thin smooth cortex with empty lumen.

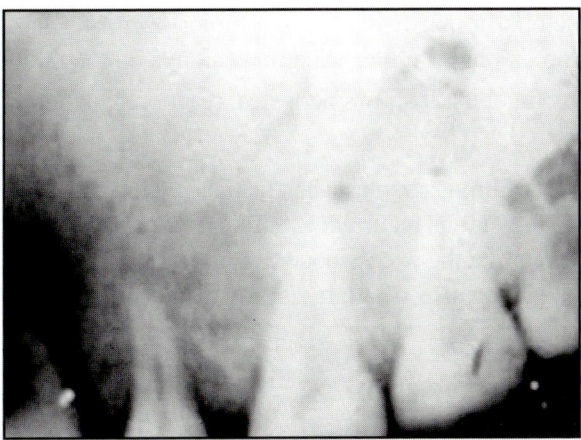

Fig. 16.3: IOPA radiograph showing orange peel appearance of fibrous dysplasia.

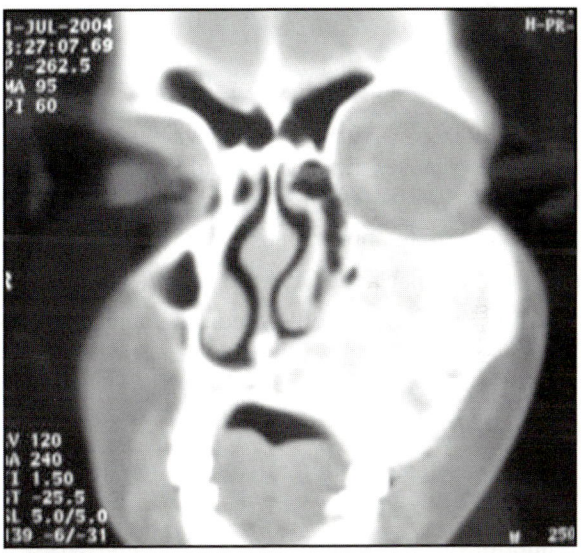

Fig. 16.4: CT scan showing opacification of sinus due to fibrous dysplasia

2. PCD/Cementoma: The age, site and the presence of a radiolucent capsule in PCD serve to differentiate it from FD.

3. Reparative giant cell granuloma: It has thin well-defined cortex, and usually occurs in the anterior jaw and has an unrestricted growth potential.

4. Ameloblastoma: It is a benign tumor occurring in an older age group and has a multilocular appearance on the radiograph.
5. Osteomyelitis: It shows periosteal reaction which is absent in FD.

Treatment

The treatment of fibrous dysplasia can be delayed until the somatic growth is complete to prevent its recurrence. Surgical recontouring/shaving can be performed to remove the excess bone. Radiotherapy may be effective, but contraindicated because of high risk of transforming the lesion into osteosarcoma.

CHERUBISM

Cherubism, also known as familial fibrous dysplasia is a rare inherited disorder causing bilateral enlargement of the jaws. It is called as cherubism because it gives the patient a *Cherub*, i.e. *angel* like appearance.

Clinical Features

 (i) Children present with painless swelling of the lower face.
 (ii) At times, there may be a profound swelling of the maxilla.
 (iii) This swelling causes the lower eyelid to be retracted exposing the sclera of the lower part of the eye with the *'Eyes raised to the heaven'* kind of an appearance.
 (iv) The submandibular nodes may be enlarged and palpable.
 (v) Syndromes such as Ramon's syndrome and Noonan's syndrome may be associated with cherubism.

Radiographic Features

 (a) It appears as large, bilateral, multilocular, expansile lesion (Fig. 16.5).
 (b) The interior of the lesion shows fine granular wispy trabeculae.
 (c) The tooth buds may be destroyed or characteristically displaced anteriorly.
 (d) The lesions may show signs of regression and by late adulthood, the bone may appear to be completely normal.

D.D.

The main differential diagnosis for cherubism include Giant cell granuloma but mainly occurs anterior to the first molar and multiple OKC,

Gorlin-Goltz syndrome in which teeth are displaced posteriorly while they are displaced anteriorly in cherubism.

FLORID OSSEOUS DYSPLASIA (FOD)

(i) This term was coined by Melrose et al in which normal cancellous bone is replaced by acellular cemento-osseous tissue.

(ii) The term florid means extensive/widespread. The lesions are multifocal lesions in all quadrants.

(iii) Middle-aged black females are usually affected. The mandible is commonly affected than the maxilla.

(iv) FOD is usually painless and may cause expansion of the jaws.

(v) There may be a complaint of a dull aching pain with sinus discharge, but the teeth in the affected region remain vital.

(vi) Mucosal ulceration on the surface can lead to osteomyelitis of the underlying bone.

Radiographic Appearance

(a) Multiple mixed radiolucent-radiopaque lesions are seen bilaterally (Fig. 16.6).

(b) Multiple simple bone cysts may be present in the jaws that appear as periapical radiolucencies. They are formed due to obstruction to the drainage of normal interstitial fluid by the fibro-osseous proliferation.

(c) Hypercementosis of the roots may be present in some cases.

(d) Large masses can cause inferior displacement of canal or superior displacement of floor of sinus.

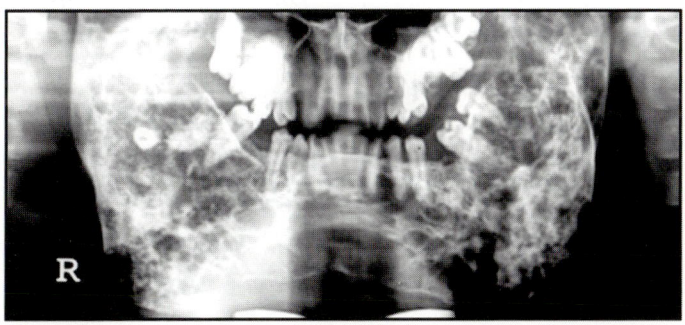

Fig. 16.5: OPG showing large multilocular lesion of cherubism in the mandible.

D.D.: Includes Paget's disease, polyostotic FD, osteomyelitis and secondary osteomyelitis in FOD.

Treatment of choice is removal of the cemental masses and curettage.

OSSIFYING FIBROMA

It is a true neoplasm with significant growth potential, composed of fibrous tissue containing a mixture of admixed bony trabeculae, cementum like spherules or both.

Clinical Features

   (i) It presents as slow growing painless expansion of the jaw and occurs only in the facial bone.

 (ii) The mandible is more commonly affected than the maxilla.

(iii) They are frequently found in the premolar-molar region, above the canal.

(iv) The juvenile form of this disease is quite aggressive and affects the 1st and 2nd decade of life.

 (v) It is a very well-defined lesion and separates out easily from the remaining bone at surgery.

(vi) Tooth displacement is an early sign in this disease.

Radiographic Features

(a) Ossifying fibroma may appear as well-defined mixed lesion with a radiolucent capsule around it.

(b) Occasionally, it may be radiolucent with few radiopaque flecks of trabeculae within the lesion.

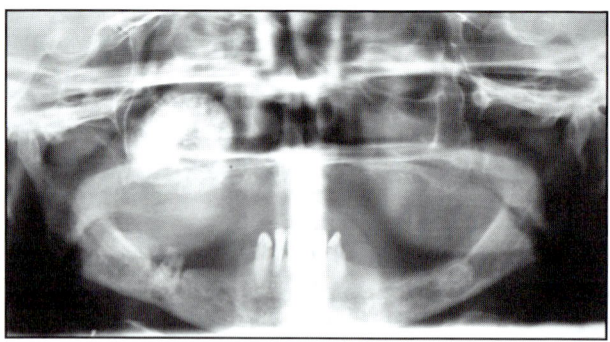

Fig. 16.6: OPG showing large cemental masses of FOD in the maxilla and mandible.

(c) Expansion and thinning of cortical plates is a characteristic finding.

(d) Displacement of teeth and canal is also noted in several cases. However, root resorption is rare.

D.D. includes fibrous dysplasia, osteosarcoma, CEOT, CEOC, etc.

Treatment involves surgical enucleation of the lesion. Larger lesions may have to be resected. As quoted by H.M.Worth, fibrous dysplasia is a condition of the bone, but ossifying fibroma is a tumor in bone.

PAGET'S DISEASE

It is also known as osteitis deformans and characterized by abnormal resorption and apposition of bone. There occurs an intense wave of osteoclastic resorption resulting in irregular cavities in the bone which is followed by vigorous osteoblastic activity.

Clinical Features

(i) It is essentially a disease of old age characterize by slow expansion of the jaws. Denture wearing patients may complain of a feeling of tightness of dentures.

(ii) Bone pain may be sometimes significant. Neuralgic pain may be present due to narrowing of the foramina through which the nerves pass.

(iii) Gradual separation of the teeth takes place causing malocclusion.

(iv) Other bones such as sacrum, pelvis, femur, skull and vertebra may also be affected.

(v) S.Alkaline phosphatase and urine hydroxyproline levels are raised which signify rapid turnover of bone.

Radiographic Features

(a) During the early resorptive stage the lesion appears radiolucent.

(b) Later on it may acquire a mixed stage which presents with a granular ground glass appearance.

(c) The trabeculae are reduced in number, long and arranged in a horizontal linear pattern.

(d) In the advanced stages, there appear rounded radiopaque patches within the bone which have a *cotton wool* appearance.

(e) Patients may have a prominent Pagetoid skull which is 3–4 times thicker than normal.

(f) The jaws are elongated with thinning of cortices.

(g) The overall density of jaw is increased.

(h) In some cases, there may be generalized hypercementosis.

(i) Areas of bone lysis may be seen as well-defined radiolucencies in the skull bones and are known as osteoporosis circumscripta.

Paget's disease is treated with calcitonin and sodium etidronate that help to reduce the osteoclastic activity and pain. The complications include delayed healing of extraction socket, osteomyelitis and osteosarcoma.

Important Differentiating Features between Fibrous Dysplasia and Osteomyelitis

Fibrous dysplasia	Osteomyelitis
Margins blend imperceptibly	The lesion has permeative margins
Fingerprint pattern may be seen on radiographs	A stippled bone pattern may be seen on the radiographs.
Expansion of cortex and displacement of sinus wall occurs	Perpendicular spiculations and periosteal reactions are seen
The lamina dura - imperceptible because of osseous changes and there occurs narrowing of periodontal ligament space	Destruction of lamina dura and Widening of periodontal ligament space are noted
Smooth blending margins	The margins are irregular with radiolucent periphery
Granular/fingerprint appearance of the bone	Sequestrum formation may be evident on the radiograph as radiopaque mass
Cortex appears displaced and ribbon like	The original cortex is preserved within the expansion
Periosteal reactions are not seen	Periosteal reactions may be seen

CHAPTER 17

Advanced Imaging Modalities for Maxillofacial Region

XERORADIOGRAPHY

Xeroradiography is a technique in which a charged selenium plate is used as an image recording device. When exposed to radiation, the selenium plate loses the charge in the areas that have received radiation. The exposed plate is then processed in a special processor to obtain a positive image with the exposed areas appearing light and the unexposed areas appearing dark (blue). The image is then fixed on a paper and becomes ready to be viewed under reflected light.

The advantages of Xeroradiography are:

1. No wet processing is involved.
2. Images with high resolution (up to **200 line pairs per mm**) can be obtained.
3. Xeroradiography provides high exposure latitude.
4. No special illumination or viewing devices are required.
5. *Edge enhancement:* The margins between the radiolucent and radiopaque structures appear clear, thereby making fine details apparent.
6. Xeroradiography provides excellent soft tissue details and is found to be useful in mammography.

ULTRASONOGRAPHY (USG)

USG is a modality that uses sound waves for imaging. These ultrasonic sound waves have a high frequency and are not audible to the human ear.

Principle

Sound travels at different speeds in different materials. In other words, each material has its own acoustic impedance. In USG, the sound waves are directed at an object. These waves strike the different layers of the object and are reflected back. The reflected waves carry information regarding the object which can be visualized on a specialized device/ TV screen/ photographic plate.

Indications

USG has a limited role in maxillofacial radiology and is used to study salivary gland pathology, lymph nodes, carotid calcification and blood flow patterns, etc. It is widely used in echocardiography and in obstetrics to study the fetus.

COMPUTED TOMOGRAPHY SCANS (CT SCANS)

CT scans were introduced by Godfrey Hounsfield in 1970. Computerized tomography is a type of cross sectional tomography in which all unwanted planes or layers of the body are completely eliminated using mathematical technique (Fig. 17.1). The basic apparatus of a CT works much on the principles as a dental tomography machine. A gantry is used to support the X-ray source located directly opposite to a bank of radiation detectors that measure the attenuation of the X-ray beam. The part of the patient's body to be scanned is interposed between the X-ray source and the detectors and a series of exposures are made over an arc of 180° to 360° with the X-ray beam collimated to determine the thickness of the slice. When the full series of view are obtained, the patient is moved and contiguous areas are scanned. The images thus obtained are sent to a computer and processed.

CT scans are indicated to study space occupying lesions in the brain, evaluation of trauma in head injury cases (Fig. 17.2). They are excellent for studying the localization, extension and nature of pathologies of the jaws. Modified CT scan called denta scan is ideal for pre-implant assessment. With the introduction of contrast media it is possible to diagnose soft tissue pathologies.

CONE BEAM COMPUTED TOMOGRAPHY SCAN (CBCT)

CBCT stands for cone beam computed tomography. It differs from CT in the fact that it uses cone-shaped beam as opposed to fan-shaped beam of X-rays in CT. To obtain images CT requires multiple rotation of this fan-shaped beam in helical fashion but as CBCT uses cone-shaped beam the area to be imaged can be covered in single 360 degrees rotation of the machine around patient .This significantly reduces time required for image acquisition. Also reduction in the number of rotations of X-ray beam reduces

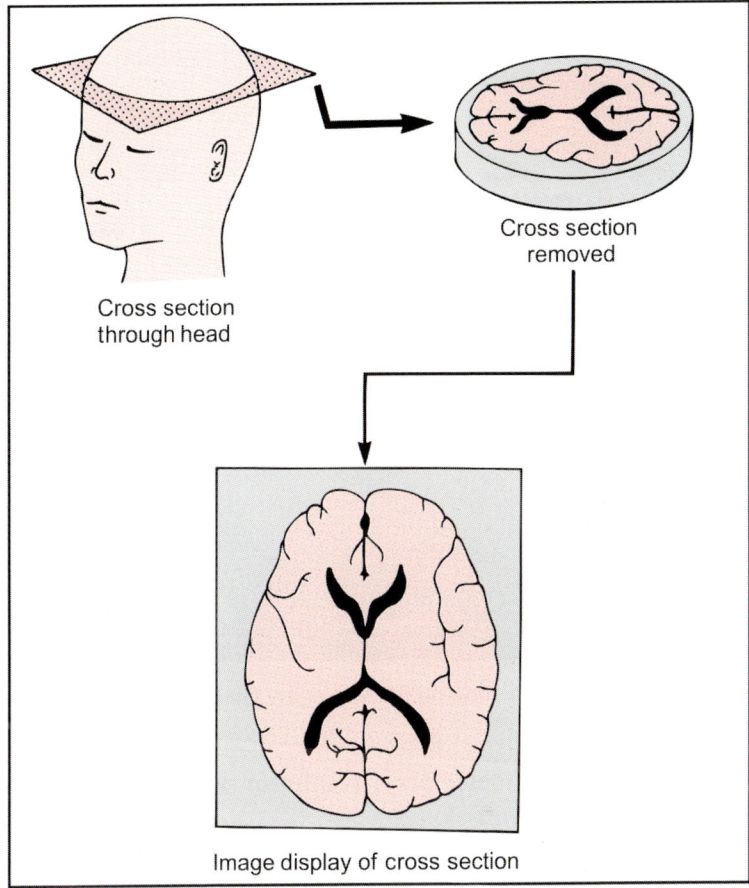

Cross section
removed

Cross section
through head

Image display of cross section

Fig. 17.1: Diagram showing the principle of CT scan.

radiation exposure to patient. Moreover CBCT allows collimation of X-beam only to the area of interest (i.e. Field of View) which further enhances benefit of reduced radiation exposure to patient.

Like CT scan CBCT also provides 3-D reconstruction of images. This reconstruction in CT depends on thickness of slice used while taking scan while in CBCT it depends on Pixels in the area of detector.

Advantages

1. Rapid scanning time [CBCT = less than 30 sec]
2. Reduced radiation exposure to patient [CBCT= 52–1025 μSv , CT= 1400–2100 μSv]

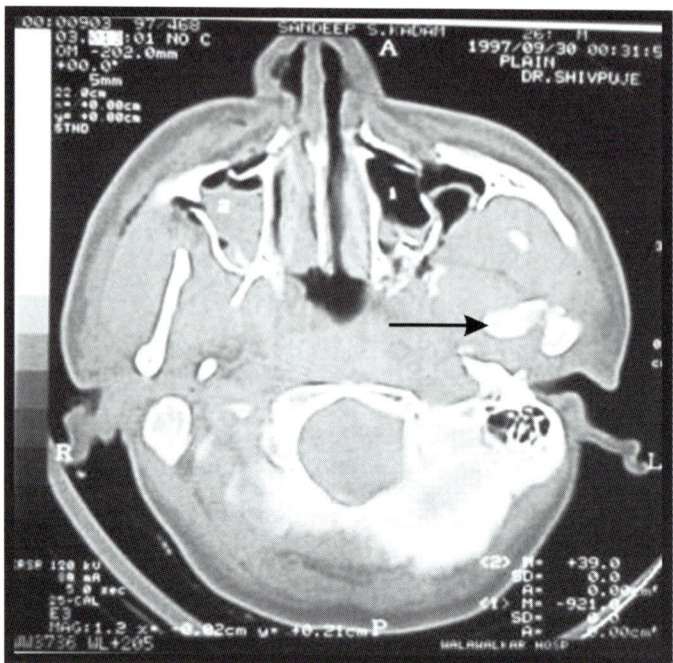

Fig. 17.2: CT scan showing fracture of the left condyle (arrow).

3. It provides sub-millimeter pixel resolution which is required for maxillofacial imaging.
4. Interactive display modes available in CBCT by using its special software allows its multifold use in dentistry.

Disadvantages

They mainly are due to cone-shaped geometry of beam

1. Grainy image
2. Areas which are present in central portion of beam are better recorded than the areas in the peripheral portion of the beam as in this portion of X-ray beam is less attenuated.
3. Streak artifacts which are seen due to metallic restorations are more pronounced.
4. Due to poor soft tissue contrast CBCT is useful only for hard tissue imaging.
5. With the help of contrast enhancement it is possible to detect soft tissue details with CT scan such as peripheral enhancement in abscess and

central enhancement in tumors with greater vascularity, such a facility is not available with present CBCT.

Uses

1. Presurgical assessment for implant placement and for disimpactions cases
2. To assess bony pathologies of maxillofacial region
3. For imaging of Temporomandibular joint pathologies
4. To obtain 3-Dimensional image of root canals
5. To assess dental pathologies.

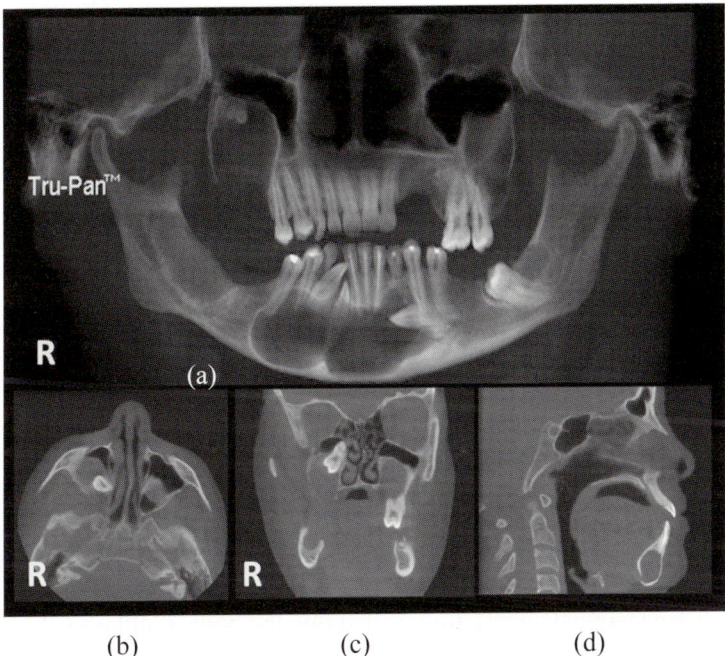

Fig. 17.3: CBCT Scan: (a)Tru-Pan view showing multiple cysts involving the mandible and maxilla,(b) Axial view showing impacted tooth and associated cyst in the right side maxillary sinus,(c) Coronal view showing impacted tooth and cysts involving both right and left maxillary sinuses and right side mandible,(d) Sagittal view showing cyst involving the mandible.

MAGNETIC RESONANCE IMAGING (MRI)

In MRI scans, the patient is placed in a strong magnetic field which causes alignment of the H^+ ions in the body in a particular direction. Radio waves of high frequency are directed towards the object at right angles. This gives rise to H$^+$ ion spin. The H$^+$ ions which have rotated take some time to return to their original position and to realign themselves. During this time, certain impulses are given out which are detected by special devices and sent to a computer which generates the image.

Advantages of MRI Scans

   i. Since H$^+$ ions are concentrated in the soft tissue, MRI scan provides excellent soft tissue contrast and hence can be used to study CNS pathology, meniscus of the TMJ, salivary glands, etc.

  ii. The absence of ionizing radiation makes it safer for use.

 iii. Direct sagittal sections can be obtained unlike in CT where these sections have to be reconstructed.

     However, MRI scans require a long time for image acquisition and hence patient cooperation is required during the procedure. Also patients with severe claustrophobia and those having cardiac pacemakers or aneurysmal clips cannot be subjected to MRI scanning (Fig. 17.4).

Indications for MRI

1. To study soft tissue pathologies such as CNS pathology, malignancies and other tumors involving the tongue, floor of the mouth, pharynx.
2. To study lymph nodes and space infections.
3. To study salivary gland pathologies.
4. To study TMJ pathologies mainly internal disc derangement and effusion.

SCINTIGRAPHY

It is mainly indicated for whole body scanning to detect metastasis. Scintigraphy/radioisotope scanning is a procedure in which radiopharmaceutical agents are injected into the body. Unlike a CT scan or MRI, which record anatomical changes, scintigraphy detects and records the functional changes taking place within the lesion. The agents accumulate at the disease sites and emit radiation which can be detected by special scintillation cameras and converted into image suitable for viewing, e.g. malignant neoplasm with high cellular activity will concentrate more of the radiopharmaceutical and will appear as a hotspot on the scintigraph (Fig. 17.5).

     The commonly used radiopharmaceutical agents are gallium 67, technetium pertechnate 99m, iodine131, etc.

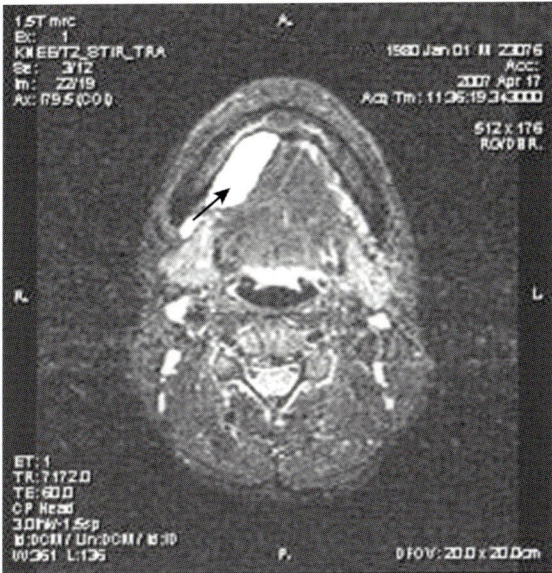

Fig. 17.4: MRI scan showing a hyperintense vascular lesion in the floor of the mouth (arrow).

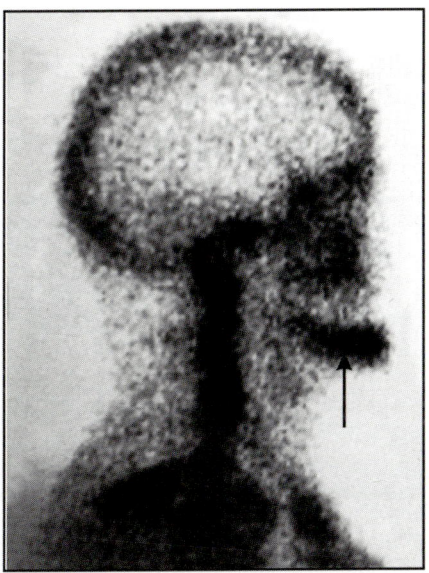

Fig. 17.5: Scintigram showing increased uptake of tracer (hot-spot) in the mandible suggestive of a tumor (arrow).

FUSION IMAGING (HYBRID IMAGING)

It is observed that even if scintigraphy shows functional changes taking place within the body, it fails to define the exact anatomical location of the lesion. The evolution of fused PET-CT/MRI also known as hybrid imaging is particularly promising since it combines the advantage of detailed imaging of the anatomy combined with detection of local metabolic activity pattern. Hence for the first time this technique offers simultaneous direct information of anatomy and physiological function of bone pathology. The ultimate purpose of image fusion is to impose a structural anatomic framework on functional images (Fig. 17.6).

Advantages

i. Providing structural and functional information in the same image
ii. Improving reading efficiency
iii. Improving confidence in diagnosis when one modality alone is not definitive
iv. Quantification of the difference between scans.

Applications

i. Evaluation of cancer
ii. Radiation therapy planning
iii. Quantification of therapy response

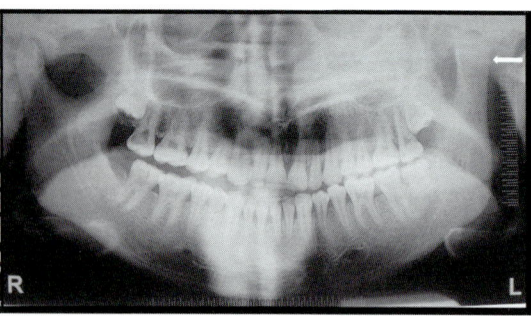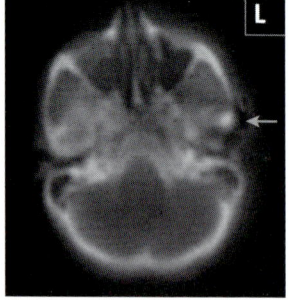

Fig. 17.6: OPG showing left condylar hyperplasia and the fusion image showing increased uptake in the left condylar region.

SUGGESTED READING AND REFERENCES

1. Oral Radiology. Principles and Interpretation: White & Pharoah - 6th edition.

2. Essentials of Dental Radiography and Radiology. Eric Whaites, 3rd edition.

3. A Guide to Dental Radiography—Rita Mason, Sarah Whaites, 3rd edition.

4. Panoramic Radiology. Langland.

5. Principles and Practice of Oral Radiographic Interpretations. H.M.Worth.

6. Contemporary Dental and Maxillofacial Imaging DCNA October 2008.

Notes

Radiographic Differential Diagnosis

When presented with an abnormal looking Radiographic appearance an effort is made to understand and explain such an appearance.

If the unusual appearance is bilaterally symmetrical and patient is not having any signs or symptoms the possibility of anatomic variation is considered. If there is a clearcut evidence of a lesion on the radiograph, clinical and radiographic correlation is carried out and a provisional diagnosis is made.

Quite often it is felt that there may be two or more lesions which may have a similar clinical and radiographic presentation and therefore a list of Differential Diagnosis is made and further logical reasoning and investigations are carried out to pinpoint the accurate diagnosis. Even if it is well established that the final diagnosis is given by the pathologist, the radiologist must make every effort to exercise his acumen and utilize his knowledge and experience to differentially diagnose various lesions.

A very concise list of **Differential Diagnosis** of various radiographic appearances is presented below:

1. Periapical Radiolucency

i. *Normal variation:* Mental foramen, incisive foramen

ii. *Periapical cyst:* Smooth, round, continuous, corticated, size: more than 1.6 cm

iii. *Periapical granuloma:* Smooth, round, continuous, non-corticated, size : less than 1.6 cm

iv. *Periapical abscess:* Ill-defined radiolucency

v. *Periapical cemental dysplasia (PCD):* In early stage there is somewhat rounded radiolucency with well-defined borders and associated with teeth having vital pulps

  vi. *Buccal bifurcation cyst:* Circular, corticated radiolucency centered a little distal to the furcation of the involved tooth, most commonly the permanent mandibular first molar.

  vii. *Periodontal abscess:* Diffuse radiolucency seen associated with excessive bone loss

  viii. *Osteomyelitis:* Ill-defined radiolucency with ragged borders (moth-eaten appearance) and sequestrae within the radiolucency

  ix. *Carcinoma:* Area of radiolucency with ragged and ill-defined permeative borders (bays and promontories like appearance), floating or hanging teeth and spiked root resorption

2. Pericoronal Radiolucency

  i. *Dentigerous cyst:* Well demarcated and corticated margins attached to the cementoenamel junction of the associated tooth

  ii. *Odontogenic keratocyst:* Large multilocular radiolucency with well corticated margins commonly seen at the mandibular posterior region, at times crossing the midline. Relatively less superior or inferior border expansion compared to ameloblastoma.

  iii. *Adenomatoid odontogenic tumor:* Common in maxillary anterior region, appears as well-defined radiolucency with small radiopaque flecks within (Milky Way lumen appearance), lesion covers greater portion of the tooth beyond CE Junction

  iv. *Ameloblastic fibroma:* Unilocular or multilocular pericoronal radiolucency, closely resembles dentigerous cyst, may show cortical expansion, a common location is near the crest of the alveolar process.

  v. *Ameloblastoma:* Mural or unicystic ameloblastoma—a pericoronal radiolucency with scalloped borders and septa or trabeculae within.

3. Multilocular Lesions

  i. *Ameloblastoma:* Soap bubble or honeycomb appearance, coarse and curved septa seen, blunt root resorption, tooth displacement is common, superior or inferior border expansion.

  ii. *Odontogenic keratocyst:* Large multilocular radiolucency with well corticated margins. Tends to extend along the marrow spaces causing less expansion.

  iii. *Aneurysmal bone cyst:* Unilocular or multilocular radiolucency with demarcated borders.

iv. *Odontogenic myxoma:* Well defined multilocular lesion with internal structure made of thin, straight bony trabeculae arranged at right angle to the periphery (tennis racket appearance).

v. *Calcifying epithelial odontogenic cyst*: Multilocular radiolucency with areas of calcification within, most commonly seen anterior to first molars in maxilla and mandible

vi. *Haemangioma:* Multilocular radiolucency with radial arrangement of trabeculae (spokes of wheel appearance).

vii. *Cherubism:* Large, bilateral, multilocular, expansile lesion. Tooth buds may be destroyed or characteristically displaced anteriorly. Small, medium and large sized locules coexist

viii. *Central giant cell granuloma:* Multilocular radiolucency most commonly seen in the region anterior to mandibular first molar and crossing the midline. Interior of the lesion shows fine, granular, wispy trabeculae.

4. Unilocular Lesions Tooth Associated : Periapical /Pericoronal

5. Lesions Separate from Tooth

i. *Traumatic bone cyst:* Periapical radiolucency with intact lamina dura of the teeth in the same region. Cystic radiolucency is well-defined above the mandibular canal and extends superiorly between the roots of premolars and molars producing scalloped appearance

ii. *Static bone cyst/Stafne's cyst/Lingual mandibular bone defect:* Radiolucency surrounded by a smooth, dense radiopaque rim which is ovoid or round in shape, usually unilocular but can be bilocular also. Located inferior to the mandibular canal in the third molar region. Sialography performed to confirm that it is anatomically the submandibular gland fossa.

iii. *Incisive canal cyst/ nasopalatine cyst:* Cystlike radiolucency projected over the apices of maxillary central incisors. Often the anterior nasal spine is seen over the superior portion of the cyst as a radiopaque shadow, thus producing a heart-shaped radiolucency

iv. *Globulomaxillary cyst:* Inverted pear or tear-shaped, well-defined radiolucency between the separated roots of the lateral incisor and canine. Careful examination reveals that the lamina dura around the roots of both teeth is intact.

6. Irregular Radiolucencies

i. *Carcinoma:* Area of radiolucency with ragged and ill-defined permeative borders (bays and promontories like appearance), floating or hanging teeth and spiked root resorption. Frank destruction of the anatomic landmarks, e.g. inferior dental canal, walls of the maxillary antrum.

ii. *Abscess:* Ill-defined radiolucency associated with a carious tooth or bone loss (periodontal).

iii. *Osteomyelitis:* Ill-defined radiolucency with ragged borders (moth-eaten appearance) and sequestra within the radiolucency and periosteal bone formation (involucrum).

iv. *Osteoradionecrosis:* History of radiotherapy, large sequestra, pathological fracture and absence of periosteal reaction.

v. *Osteosarcoma:* Radiolucency with poorly defined, ragged borders. Bandlike widening involving the complete length of the periodontal ligament space on one or both sides of the root (Garrington's sign). Epicenter within the body of the mandible, possibility of pathological fracture. Commonly associated with periosteal reactions, classically sunburst appearance.

vi. *Multiple myeloma:* Multiple, separate, well-defined, non-corticated lesions (punched out).

vii. *Metastatic carcinoma:* Moderately well-demarcated, non-corticated, polymorphous in shape and may have ill-defined invasive margins.

viii. *Eosinophilic granuloma:* Multiple, well-defined radiolucencies with faint ragged borders in juveniles and definitive radiolucencies with some sclerosing borders in adults. The alveolar process is frequently involved in lesions that involve bone superior to the mandibular canal.

7. Floating Tooth

i. *Periodontitis/Periodontal abscess:* Here the associated alveolar bone loss is parallel to the original lamina dura and there is peripheral condensation of bone as a reaction to infective process.

ii. *Carcinoma:* Associated alveolar bone loss is highly irregular and there is no peripheral condensation of bone, roots show spiked resorption

iii. *Osteomyelitis:* Presents as an irregular area of osteolysis surrounding the roots, sequestra and periosteal reaction are also seen.

iv. *Cherubism:* Multilocular radiolucency appearing bilaterally in the jaws giving rise to displacement of the teeth.

v. *Eosinophilic granuloma:* Presents as a saucer-shaped or a scooped out osteolytic lesion surrounding the roots of the teeth and often manifested bilaterally.

8. Radiopaque Lesions

i. *Bone:*

a. *Periapical Cemental Dysplasia:* Well-defined, crescentic radiopacity apical to the roots surrounded by a radiolucent halo

b. *Cementoblastoma:* Rare lesion seen as a well-defined radiopacity attached to the root/s, surrounded by a radiolucent capsule and a corticated border outside it.

c. *Condensing osteitis:* Radiopacity surrounds the radiolucency around the root apex, trabeculae can be visualized within the radiopacity.

d. *Enostosis:* Radiopaque dense bone island present within the bone without any radiolucent margin, occasionally blends with the trabeculae of the surrounding bone.

e. *Exostosis:* Well-defined and smoothly contoured, homogenously radiopaque lesion with curved border which presents as a bony projection.

f. *Osteoma:* Well-defined, uniformly radiopaque. Can be of three types: Cancellous (bone marrow spaces visible), compact (uniformly opaque like ivory), osteoid (with a radiolucent nidus)

ii. Tooth-like:

a. Supernumerary tooth

b. *Odontome:* As odontome is made up of dental tissues, its radiopacity is equal to that of a tooth.

Compound: Multiple teeth-like structures (denticles) having enamel, dentine, etc. and surrounded by a fibrous capsule.

Complex: Single, dense radiopaque mass surrounded by a radiolucent fibrous capsule (enamel and dentine cannot be distinguished).

c. *Fibro-odontome*

iii. *Miscellaneous:*

a. *Sialolith:* Commonly seen in Wharton's duct as a whorled or uniform radiopacity.

b. *Lymph node calcification:* At times presents as a radiopacity resembling cauliflower. Patient may give history of tuberculosis.

c. *Phlebolith:* Multiple separate radiopacities associated with vascular lesions having a concentric appearance with a radiolucent centre (bulls eye).

d. Antrolith: Radiopacity seen within the antrum.

e. Rhinolith

f. Tonsillolith

g. *Vessel wall calcification:* Pipe stem/tram track appearance.

h. *Eagle's syndrome:* Metastatic calcification of the stylohyoid ligament.

i. *Cysticercosis:* Multiple, elliptical radiopacities (tapeworm infestation).

j. *AOT:* Multiple, small flecks of calcification seen within the tumor

k. *CEOT:* Multiple, scattered radiopacities close to the crown of the embedded tooth.

9. Mixed Radiolucent-Radiopaque Lesions

i. *Ossifying fibroma/ Cement-ossifying fibroma:* Well-defined mixed lesion with a radiolucent capsule around it.

ii. *Florid osseous dysplasia:* Mixed radiolucent-radiopaque lesions are seen bilaterally and present in both the jaws (cotton wool appearance)

iii. *Fibrous dysplasia:* Periphery of the lesion is ill-defined with a gradual blending of normal trabecular bone into an abnormal trabecular pattern. Various appearances seen are ground glass, orange peel and fingerprint.

Radiographic Appearances

Descriptive term for radiographic appearance	Condition/s
Soap bubble, Honey comb, spider-web like appearance	Ameloblastoma
Strings of tennis racket appearance	Odontogenic myxoma
Hair on end appearance	Thalassemia, sickle cell anemia
Copper beaten skull/ digital markings	Crouzon's syndrome
Arnold head/ Light bulb skull	Cleidocranial dysplasia
Geographic skull	Hand-Schüller-Christian disease
Pepper pot skull	Hyperparathyroidism
Apple core appearance	Radiation induced caries
Orange peel appearance/ peau d'orange	Fibrous dysplasia
Ground-glass appearance	Fibrous dysplasia, hyperparathyroidism, ossifying fibroma
Thumb print appearance	Fibrous dysplasia
Onion skin/onion peel appearance	Garre's osteomyelitis, osteosarcoma, Ewing's sarcoma
Cotton wool appearance	Paget's disease, fibrous dysplasia
Rib within rib appearance	Thalassemia
Milky Way lumen	AOT
Step ladder appearance	Sickle cell anemia, odontogenic myxoma, normal trabecular pattern
Chicken wire appearance	Thalassemia
Moth-eaten appearance	Osteomyelitis
Bays and promontories	Carcinoma
Ghost teeth	Regional odontodysplasia
Thistle tube shaped pulp chamber	Dentine dysplasia
Salt and pepper appearance– Radiographic	Thallasemia
Salt and pepper appearance – MRI	Sjögren's syndrome
Bow-tie appearance	Normal interarticular disc in MRI
Gumball appearance	Anterior disc displacement in MRI

Toadstool appearance	Juvenile arthritis/ Boering's arthrosis
Sharpened pencil appearance	Rheumatoid arthritis
Trapdoor /Bright light sign	Blow out fracture
Sunray/ sunburst appearance	Osteosarcoma, chondrosarcoma, central Haemangioma
Tramline calcification	Sturge-Weber syndrome
Spokes of wheel appearance	Central haemangioma, healing periapical cyst
Donut appearance	Healing periapical cyst
Coming through donut appearance	Dentigerous cyst
Spiked roots	Malignancy
Joint mice	Osteoarthritis
Codman's triangle	Osteosarcoma
Garrington's sign	Osteosarcoma
Tyre track appearance	Reverse placement of the film
Pipe stem/ tram track appearance	Arteriosclerosis
Bulls eye appearance	Dilacerated root, lingually impacted third molars
Driven snow appearance	Pindborg tumor
Peripheral cuffing	Peripheral giant cell granuloma
Elephant trunk appearance	Normal appearance of the zygoma in PA Water's view
Cumulus cloud appearance	Osteosarcoma

Sialographic appearances

Leafless tree	Normal sialographic appearance
Tree in winter	Normal sialographic appearance of parotid gland
Bush in winter	Normal sialographic appearance of submandibular gland
Branchless fruit laden tree/ Cherry blossom	Sjögren's syndrome
Snow storm appearance	Sjögren's syndrome
Apple tree like appearance	Sialadenitis
Filling defect	Sialolithiasis
Sausage string appearance	Sialodochitis
Saccular enlargement	Sialodochitis
Ball in hand appearance	Benign tumor
Puddling and pooling of contrast media	Intrinsic invasive tumor

Index